NURSIN
GENERA

The to kit f
hea th ca

2015

poell
gbottom
nd
son Po

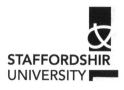

STAFFORDSHIR
UNIVERSITY

orking in Partnership
ogramme

Radcliffe Publishing Ltd
18 Marcham Road
Abingdon
Oxon OX14 1AA
United Kingdom

www.radcliffe-oxford.com
Electronic catalogue and worldwide online ordering facility.

British Library Cataloguing in Publication Data

A catalogue record for this book is available from the British Library.

ISBN-13: 978 1 84619 172 5

Typeset by Phoenix Photosetting, Chatham, Kent
Printed and bound by TJ International Ltd, Padstow, Cornwall

Contents

Preface

This book has been commissioned by the NHS Working in Partnership Programme (WiPP).

We are delighted to have worked with the authors to bring you a valuable resource that will support general practice. It will help you to extend and enhance the role that nurses and health care assistants (HCAs) play in delivering high-quality care to patients.

There are already over 300 million consultations in primary care, and this number is set to increase because of the shift of care from the acute sector to primary care. It is therefore vital that general practice, being the hub of primary care, is sufficiently staffed and skilled to take on this challenge.

The Health Care Assistant Initiative and General Practice Nursing Initiative aim to support the development of nurses and HCAs employed in general practice in order to:

- improve patient care
- create a rewarding environment for nurses and HCAs in general practice
- make working in general practice an attractive career option.

This book is based on the Web-based toolkits developed as part of the General Practice Nursing and HCA WiPP Initiatives. You can access these toolkits by visiting www.wipp.nhs.uk. This website provides the general practice team with tools and resources to employ, train, develop and enhance nurses' and HCAs' roles within the team.

With the increasing demand on primary care services, where over 90% of the population access services, it is crucial now, more than ever, that resources are used effectively. Increasingly, more complex care is being managed within general practice, and nurses are taking on more advanced roles. Inevitably this means that there is a need to encompass a greater skill mix within the nursing team. In addition, the dawning of practice-based commissioning (PBC) means that there are further new opportunities for nurses working in general practice. In order for nurses to be able to advance their skills and roles in the light of PBC, HCAs will need to feature more widely within general practice and take on a range of tasks that have hitherto been performed by qualified nurses.

Nursing in general practice is a relatively new career option for nurses and HCAs. This book, together with the development of a general practice nursing career framework and resources from the WiPP website, raises awareness of career possibilities. It encourages practices to further develop and support their nursing staff and plan for opportunities that will develop skills at all levels, in order to ensure a practice team that is working at maximum capability.

We trust that you will find this resource useful.

Sue Cross
National Project Manager
General Practice Nursing Initiative
Working in Partnership Programme

Paul Vaughan
National Project Manager
Health Care Assistants Initiative
Working in Partnership Programme

May 2007

The Working in Partnership Programme

The NHS is a dynamic organisation that is constantly reshaping itself to meet the health care needs of people living in a modern world. Change is an integral part of the process required to keep the NHS relevant and fit for purpose. Change can be challenging and yet provide exciting opportunities to develop new ways of working focused on the people using the service.

General practice has not been immune from the challenges facing the NHS in the current complex health care environment. Some of the challenges facing general practice include:

- shortages of staff in key professional groups
- changing demographics
- the need to manage organisational costs
- a drive for patient-led services, which requires services to be built around patients
- changing health care policy – for example, *A Health Service of All the Talents* (Department of Health, 2000a), *The NHS Plan* (Department of Health, 2000b) and the NHS Changing Workforce Programme.

The Working in Partnership Programme (WiPP) was established to address some of these challenges. Born out of the new GMS Contract (2003), it aims to support general practice to proactively manage the future needs of the service and ensure that it is in a position to adapt to the rapidly changing face of health care in the future. WiPP sets out to create capacity in general practice in two ways:

1. by reducing the public's need for general practice services through improved self-care
2. by developing new ways of working that improve efficiency.

To assist with reducing the public's need for general practice services, WiPP has developed a range of self-care resources to support self-care behaviours among the public, through healthy living, minor ailments management and management of long-term conditions. To promote new ways of working, WiPP is developing initiatives that will redirect demand for services outside general practice, substitute workload within general practice and increase efficiency in general practice.

There are 13 WiPP initiatives, each of which contributes to meeting the aims of the programme. Details of each of these initiatives can be found on the WiPP website (www.wipp.nhs.uk).

Two initiatives that are particularly important to the development of general practice in the future are the General Practice Nursing Initiative and the Health Care Assistants Initiative.

- *General Practice Nursing – Getting it Right for Patients and Public Health –* a scheme supporting the development of general practice nursing in order to improve recruitment and retention, facilitate a broader skill mix, raise standards and minimise risk.
- *Facilitating the Employment, Training, Development and Integration of Health Care Assistants (HCAs)* – developing a package of support that will improve the understanding of the role of the HCA in general practice, encouraging recruitment, training and integration of HCAs in general practice.

Like many other health care sectors, general practice faces difficulty recruiting nurses. In addition to this, a significant number of nurses, especially those in general practice, will retire soon. The significance of these two projects should therefore not be underestimated. They will support general practice to develop roles based around patient need, and enable general practice to make the most of their workforce when addressing change in a dynamic workplace, making the most of initiatives like practice-based commissioning.

Louise Jarvis
Programme Manager
Working in Partnership Programme

Acknowledgements

The authors would particularly like to thank Paul Vaughan and Sue Cross from the Working in Partnership Programme for their contribution to the development of this book.

Our thanks also go to:

Lynda Carey, Nursing in General Practice Lead for Liverpool PCT

Dr Ruth Chambers, Professor of Primary Care, Staffordshire University, and Director of Postgraduate General Practice Education and Associate Head of Primary Care Education, West Midlands Health Authority

Gianpiero Celino, Webstar Health

Annabel Hinde, Medicom Group

Alice Smallman, Medicom Group

Alison Hughes, Primary Care Facilitator, Torfaen Local Health Board

Lynn Joels, Medicom Group

Clayre La Trobe, Director, Primary Care Operations, United Health Europe (previously WiPP Programme Manager)

Greg McConaghie, Medicom Group

Jacquie Phare, Practice Nurse Professional Lead and Nurse Practitioner (General Practice), Torbay Care Trust

Sue Reed, Clinical Consultant, Reed Associates

Matthew Rice, Independent Personal and Team Development Facilitator

Dorf Ruscoe, Senior Lecturer, General Practice Lead, Faculty of Health and Social Work, University of Plymouth

Les Storey, Principal Lecturer, University of Central Lancashire

Dr Gill Wakley, MD, freelance GP and writer

Andrea Sheldon, Heath Care Assistant, Weeping Cross Surgery, Stafford

Julie Talbot, Practice Nurse Facilitator, South Staffordshire PCT

Jane Higgs, Assistant Director, Practice-Based Commissioning, North Lancashire PCT

Staffordshire University Patients and Carers Group

GPN and HCA Initiatives Pilot Sites

Horden Group Practice, County Durham

Limes Medical Centre, Epping Forest

North Central and South Liverpool PCT

Richmond and Twickenham PCT

Ridge Medical Practice, Bradford

Southwark PCT

Thistlemoor Medical Practice, Peterborough

Torbay Care Trust

Woodlands Health Centre, Paddock Wood

Members of the Working in Partnership Programme GPN/HCA Steering Group

List of tools

About the Authors

Pam Campbell
MSc, RHV, RN, RM, PGCE
Pam has a long history of working in primary care, initially in Health Visiting and then as a practice nurse linked to public health activities. She developed to work as an advanced nurse practitioner after acquiring an MSc in Advanced Clinical Nursing (General Practice). Pam entered higher education as a senior lecturer in 1998 and has since held various roles within nurse education. She undertook a project to profile the practice nursing workforce in Shropshire and Staffordshire whilst working on secondment in the workforce development directorate of the Health Authority. She subsequently worked on projects to develop the wider community nursing workforce. Pam has been involved in nurse prescribing education for many years and led the curriculum development and delivery for extended and supplementary prescribing at Staffordshire University. She was active in lobbying for opening of the British National Formulary for Independent nurse prescribers in her role as Secretary of the Association for Nurse Prescribing (2003–2006). Pam maintains some clinical competence by working as a sexual health nurse for Stoke-on-Trent PCT for one evening per week. Her current role as development manager at Staffordshire university involves interpreting the development needs of the community health workforce.

Anne Longbottom
PGDip, MCIM
Anne began her working life in banking. After a short career break she joined a local Further Education College, where she gained experience developing learning opportunities for non-registered staff within the health and social care sectors. Before joining Staffordshire University Anne worked within the NHS to promote learning and development for staff who traditionally found it more difficult to access training opportunities. In 2005 Anne joined Staffordshire University as Project Manager for the NHS Working in Partnership Programme (WiPP) Health Care Assistant Project. She worked with the National Project Lead, PCTs and general practice staff across the country to develop a web-based toolkit to support the employment of health care assistants in general practice. Anne is currently developing a variety of courses including a Foundation Degree for non-registered professionals within health and social care.

Alison Pooler
BSc(Hons), RN, MSc
After graduating from Edinburgh university with a BSc (Hons) in Nursing Alison worked in the acute sector, in theatres, and then in Intensive Care where she remained for a number of years. She then moved into primary care to work as a practice nurse and developed an interest in respiratory care, setting up a

respiratory service and undertaking further training in many respiratory areas. She then returned to work in secondary care to take up a post as Clinical Nurse Specialist in respiratory care. During this time she became involved in teaching nurses and medical students. She now works as a senior lecturer in the Faculty of Health, Staffordshire University, and is currently in the final stages of writing up a PhD thesis on the psychological and social influences on the exacerbation rates of severe asthmatics.

1

The development of nursing and health care assistant roles in general practice

This chapter provides an introduction to the role of the nurse and the health care assistant working in general practice. It identifies the unique position for the roles and outlines the value of skill mix within general practice. It draws on national policy changes to demonstrate how the roles are changing and moving forward, and sets the context for the remaining chapters.

Contents

Introduction

General practice nursing is a relatively new branch of nursing that makes a unique contribution to patient care and has a significant part to play in the development of primary care. Nationally there are around 18,000 general practice nurses,[1] with only a small minority being employed directly by an NHS trust, and the majority being directly employed by practices. It is not known how many health care assistants work in general practice, but it thought to be a relatively small number in comparison. However, this number is likely to increase significantly in future as the importance of their role becomes recognised.

The Government White Paper entitled *Our Health, Our Care, Our Say*[2] states that 'When people are asked about their local NHS, they probably think first of their GP.' More than 90% of all patient contact takes place in primary care, and general practice offers patients and carers a point of contact for acute, routine and continuing care, and helps them to navigate through other parts of the health care system. Increasingly this includes consulting registered nurses such as nurse practitioners and practice nurses, as well as other health care professionals including physiotherapists, mental health counsellors and therapists, and non-registered staff such as health care assistants (HCAs).

General practice is facing a constant wave of new innovations, reorganisation and developments. As the number of general practitioners (GPs) and practice nurses due to retire in the next 10 years increases, new ways of working for the whole practice team will need to be considered. Across the country nurses are already developing new skills and taking on new responsibilities.[3] The nursing role in general practice already encompasses services such as health promotion, family planning, treatment room care, minor illness and the management of chronic and long-term conditions such as coronary heart disease, asthma and diabetes. As the role expands still further, it is anticipated that nurses working in extended roles will:

- complement the quality of services provided by doctors
- safely substitute for doctors in a wide array of services
- reduce the direct cost of services.

A study by Walsh and colleagues in 2003[4] examined the roles of practice nurses and found that they had:

- extended their clinical role to include diagnosis of simple and/or chronic conditions, plus their treatment and management
- developed a variety of innovative services and clinics to meet the needs of their local population
- developed a nurse triage service with a system tailored to suit the needs of the population that they serve.

The NHS Plan contained the Chief Nursing Officer's 10 key roles for nurses,[5] and these provided significant motivators for nursing in general practice to develop many new expanded roles, including nurse prescribing, diagnosis and assessment. *Modernising Nursing Careers*[6] emphasises the increasing scope for nurses to develop a structured career progression.

Registered nurses will need to relinquish some of the more task-orientated roles that they have been used to undertaking in order to take on new expanded roles. With appropriate training, health care assistants can take on many of these activities. Well-trained and supported HCAs can bring huge benefits to patient care in general practice, especially when they are well integrated within the practice team.

Nursing in general practice

The NHS Plan recognised that patients' expectations of the NHS and general practice are rising. Patients and carers want more convenient, quicker access to advice and treatment in health-related matters, and nursing has a key role to play in the delivery of patient-centred care. Many people are living longer and often have long-term or chronic illnesses that need to be managed. There is also a growing awareness among nurses of the need not only to respond to illness but also to prevent disease and promote health. Nurses working in general practice are in a position to help both opportunistically and, through planned intervention, to influence the health status of the estimated 98% of the general population who are registered with a GP.

National policies such as *The NHS Plan*,[5] *Liberating the Talents*,[7] National Service Frameworks, *Commissioning a Patient-Led NHS*[8] and the management of long-term conditions have all had an impact on the general practice role. *The NHS Plan* suggests that '... it is about working smarter to make the maximum use of the talents of all the NHS workforce.'

The changing role

There is a clear Government commitment in *Our Health, Our Care, Our Say*[2] to move what have traditionally been seen as secondary care services into primary care settings. This will have major implications for primary care teams in terms of the services they will be able to deliver. Nurses working in general practice will be critical to the success of these reforms, as they take up expanded roles in nurse prescribing, increased clinical specialisation, providing out-of-hours services or partnership responsibilities.

The primary purpose of nursing is to provide holistic health care for patients, families, carers and communities. Nurses seek to maintain all aspects of the health environment, so that it is conducive to improving health, facilitating recovery from illness or rehabilitation and, where appropriate, achieving a dignified death.[9] As nursing roles extend into areas of clinical competence that were once reserved for the medical profession, the essence of the nursing role that includes nurturing and caring could easily be lost. Health care assistants are ideally placed to provide additional support for patients in this way. The flexibility and responsiveness of general practice promote and encourage role development and autonomy which are highly valued by nurses. Indeed many nurses move into this area because they value working within a smaller clinical team. In 2002, the Wanless Report[10] emphasised that services should focus on prevention and early intervention in health care, and that people should take more responsibility for their own health and that of their families. Nurses within general practice already have, or with training and support can gain, the knowledge and skills to help to achieve this through the management of long-term conditions and encouraging self-care and self-management by patients.

Defining nursing roles

General practice nurses

The range of work performed by nurses in general practice is getting broader, and historically has developed in an ad-hoc way depending on the needs of the practice. The plethora of job titles and variety of roles is well recognised, and poses a challenge to both the profession and the NHS in terms of defining jobs and levels of practice.

The Nursing and Midwifery Council (NMC) is working to provide transparency about the standards and qualifications that are required for nursing and has, for example, agreed that higher levels of practice should constitute a recordable qualification.[11] An NHS career framework promoted by *Skills for Health*[12] has identified advanced practitioners as a distinct category (on Band 7 of the *Agenda for Change* pay structure), and as the Department of Health's *Modernising Nursing Careers Review*[13] emerges, it is expected to provide formalised guidance for career progression to identify recognised routes to advanced practice status. The Working in Partnership Programme (WiPP)[14] is striving to ensure that there is a recognised career and educational pathway for nurses working in general practice, from HCA to advanced nurse practitioner.

Blurring of medical and nursing boundaries

A study by Laurant and colleagues in 2005[15] evaluated the impact of doctor–nurse substitution in primary care by patient outcomes, process of care and resource utilisation, including cost. It found that in general there were no appreciable differences between doctors and nurses in health outcomes for patients, process of care, resource utilisation or cost. However, patient satisfaction was higher with nurse-led care, and nurses working in general practice tending to provide longer consultations, to give more information to patients and to recall patients more frequently than doctors. The impact on GPs' workload and direct costs of care was variable. The findings suggest that appropriately trained nurses can provide care of equal quality to that provided by GPs within defined areas and achieve good health outcomes for patients. However, GPs' workload may remain unchanged either because nurses are deployed to meet previously unmet needs, or because nurses generate a demand for care where previously there was none.

As primary care services develop, the need for high-quality, suitably qualified general practice nurses will continue to grow, and developing a good mix of skills at all levels within the team will be important for the safe delivery of patient care.

Health care assistants

Health care assistants (HCAs) have been in existence for many years,[16] and they represented 17% of the 1.3 million NHS workforce in 2004. HCAs work in a variety of health and social care settings, undertaking direct patient care as well as doing non-clinical work. This is most common in secondary care settings in hospitals, although HCAs are also used in community services (district nursing), and increasingly are being used in general practice. As health services move away from traditional secondary care to primary care settings, and the age of the primary care workforce continues to increase, general practice will need to consider alternative ways to cover the day-to-day work that will arise from these changes. By reviewing the skill mix and workload of their staff, practices could develop the role of the HCA, resulting in a wider range of staff with a diversity of qualifications and skills providing hands-on care for patients.

The Wanless Report 2004[17] estimated that 12.5% of the nurse's workload could be undertaken by HCAs (across all sectors), with nurse practitioners taking on 20% of the work normally undertaken by general practitioners or junior doctors. By 2020 another 144,000 HCAs will be needed to undertake tasks previously performed by practice nurses. With increased competition between health care sectors for HCAs, general practice will need to ensure that it provides a rewarding and progressive career structure for HCAs.

Information and experiences identified in the Working in Partnership

Programme (WiPP) Web-based toolkit for HCAs (www.wipp.nhs.uk) have shown that HCAs play an important role within the practice team in delivering patient care. Increasingly, appropriately trained, developed and integrated HCAs are undertaking work previously done by registered health professionals in order to meet patient and practice needs.

In the face of recent shortages, qualified staff have seen HCAs fill the gaps, providing the care that patients desperately need. More than ever, health care assistants are an essential part of the team.[18] The development of the HCA role and integration into the practice team is vital to ensure that practices are ready to participate in the service redesign and modernisation of the future primary care sector.

Scope of the HCA role

An HCA is defined as 'someone who works under the guidance of a qualified health care professional.'[12] However, this definition does not describe the variety of roles and activities undertaken by HCAs in general practice across the country. The title 'health care assistant' covers a range of roles, including nursing assistants, health care support workers and therapy assistants, depending on the health care setting in which they are working.

For example, within a hospital setting an HCA might be working on a surgical ward, helping patients with personal hygiene, making beds or taking physiological measurements, whereas a community health care assistant may be caring for patients within the patient's own home.

The role will also vary within general practice, with some health care assistants undertaking routine clinical tasks such as new patient checks and blood pressure monitoring, while others perform more complex clinical tasks, such as simple wound care and removal of sutures, and non-clinical work, including recall of patients and ordering of stock. The proportion of clinical to non-clinical work and the range of work will vary depending on the practice in which they work and its skill mix. Many practices first introduced the HCA role by encouraging reception staff to undertake some clinical tasks, such as phlebotomy.

Regulation

Registered nurses

The Nursing and Midwifery Council (NMC) *Code of Professional Conduct*[19] governs the actions of registered nurses. It emphasises the need for nurses to be aware of their level of competence, working within this to maintain professional standing and patient safety. This is important as the role of the general practice nurse expands and moves across the boundaries of nursing into medicine. The *Code of Professional Conduct* incorporates guidance on the scope of nurses' practice, which places a specific requirement on individuals to acknowledge their limits of professional competence and to undertake practice and accept responsibilities only for those activities in which they know that they are competent. If an aspect of practice is deemed to be beyond an individual's level of competence, then they must obtain help and supervision from a competent practitioner until the employer agrees that the requisite knowledge and skills have been acquired. General practice nurses cannot be required to take on a new role or task if they do not consider themselves to be competent without breaching the *Code of Professional Conduct* and being open to a charge of professional misconduct. This should always be borne in mind by employers as roles develop.

Non-registered nurses

An HCA usually works with a registered nurse who will assess their competence to undertake a task. If an HCA subsequently moves to a different general practice or the practice nurse leaves, then the assessment process may start again because the new practice or new practice nurse want to be reassured that the HCA is competent to perform to their standards. This can be both time-consuming and inefficient, and for the HCA may lead to a lack of self-confidence.

The questions of whether there should be a system of formal regulation for HCAs has been debated for some time, and *The NHS Plan*[5] committed a proposal to review the need for this. Consequently, a national consultation has explored views[20] and this has culminated in a pilot scheme of employer-led regulation for support workers. This is currently being undertaken in Scotland and, if successful, could lead to the adoption of a UK-wide employer-led approach to regulation.

Whilst this debate continues, the principles of implementing good employment practice are paramount. An effective training and assessment framework, developed in conjunction with local primary care trusts (PCTs), who also have a responsibility to ensure that general practice staff are appropriately trained, will enable HCAs to be confident in their role. Coupled with support and mentoring and the appropriate use of HCAs, this should enhance patient care. HCAs are not trained nurses but are trained in a particular role to undertake simple clinical procedures that have been taught, assessed and delegated by a registered health professional. They have a specific role to play in clinical activities within the general practice team, and should not be viewed as substitute nurses or a cheaper option for general practice. In addition, HCAs have important skills that can be used within non-clinical roles, including health promotion, administration and communication between patients and health professionals.

The Ridge Medical Practice, Bradford is a large general practice that serves around 17,500 patients and employs around 50 staff. Following on from the success of the Rapid Access Clinic, they decided to look at the work of their trained nurses. An audit showed that approximately 50% of their duties could be undertaken by someone who was appropriately trained but did not need nursing qualifications. Support, mentorship and training are provided in-house by qualified RGNs using a distance learning course run by the Primary Care Training Centre in Bradford. Competency is assessed on an annual basis and recorded in a portfolio. The HCA work covers a range of activities, namely new patient interviews, assisting at clinics, phlebotomy, electrocardiogram (ECG), blood pressure monitoring and smoking cessation. The practice has benefited in a number of ways, and the GPs and nurses have been enabled to undertake more specialised work in and out of the practice.

Complementary nursing roles: working together

There can be considerable overlap in primary care between the work of a regis-tered nurse and that of an HCA.[21] In addition, there is the newly emerging role of Assistant Practitioner,[12] which is discussed later in this chapter. Some nurses may perceive these overlaps as a threat to their role, whereas others see the overlaps as giving HCAs an opportunity to develop their role. Professional roles are changing to meet the increased patient demand for care, and as general practice nurses take on extra duties and responsibilities they will inevitably need to transfer some of their roles to their HCA colleagues as appropriate. In general, HCAs will take on task-orientated work – recognising that some of these tasks may require a high level of skill – but they will be unlikely to take on work that involves patient assessment, as this requires more detailed knowledge that is generally congruent with a registered nurse.

Clinical	Non-clinical
New patient checks	Stock control (ordering and restocking of
Height, weight, BMI checks	clinical areas)
Urinalysis	Equipment (maintenance, cleaning)
Health promotion	Summarising medical records
Blood pressure monitoring	Administrative tasks (e.g. patient recall)
Peak flow monitoring	Health promotion displays
Chaperoning	Sterilising equipment
Venepuncture	Preparation of clinical areas
Infection control	
Basic wound care	
Assisting in clinics (e.g. CDM, baby,	
well-person) **[AQ6]**	
Capillary blood tests	
Assisting in minor surgery	
Smoking cessation	
Hearing tests	
ECG recording	

Figure 1.1 The range of tasks undertaken by health care assistants in general practice

Through workforce planning and determining the desired skill mix of the practice team, the practice manager and general practice nurse lead will be able to plan and discuss with the team how the work will be appropriately shared. There needs to be a sense of unity between the nurse and the HCA for the successful fulfilment of each role.[21] This synergism can lead to development opportunities for both the HCA and the nurse (e.g. gaining skills in mentorship and supervi-sion), helping the practice to meet its business plan and achieve maximum points in the Quality and Outcomes Framework (QOF).[22]

Willow Bank Surgery, Stoke-on-Trent
The decision was taken to introduce HCAs into the integrated nursing care team in 2003. The practice decided to start with two HCAs, appointed in dual roles with a 50:50 split between HCA and receptionist duties. The idea

was that the patients would get to know the HCAs via contact with them as receptionists. Patients had already started to build relationships and trust with the HCAs in their role as receptionists, and they found it less threatening to disclose information to them in clinical situations. As a result, services were tailored more effectively to the needs of the patients and the local population.

Looking ahead

Practice-based commissioning (PBC)[23,24] provides an opportunity for practices to work together in partnership with the PCT to provide what patients want. 'GPs and other primary care professionals are in a prime position to redesign services that best meet patient needs and deliver what local people want.'[24] This means that nurses in general practice will be in a key position to help to shape local health care, based on their knowledge and experience of patient need. Practices are expected to develop a plan that states what their priorities are and how success in delivering care via PBC can be judged.[25] It is expected that patients and carers will also play an active role in the development of the plan. Practice nurses and health care assistants can provide a link between the patient and the practice and encourage patients to get involved in decision making. The role of nurses in PBC could include using a database to inform the practice about what services they should provide, based on what patients want. For example, practice nurses may be aware of patients who present with psychosexual problems, but have no appropriate service to which to refer them. Collating information on the numbers of patients requiring this service could create a cogent argument for the commissioning of a new service.

Progression of the nursing role in general practice

Routes for progression for both HCAs and registered nurses in general practice are now beginning to emerge. The WiPP Web-based toolkits (www.wipp.nhs.uk) provide guidance on career progression and the multiple factors that need to be considered. *Skills for Health*[12] also provides a clear outline structure for career progression.

Health care assistants

For HCAs, gaining National Vocational Qualifications (NVQs) at Further Education colleges demonstrates competence at certain levels. Achievement of NVQ level 3 is a recognised route to a higher education diploma or degree in nursing if an HCA wanted to move into registered nurse training. However, not all HCAs want to take this route, and many will be content to carry on in their current general practice role. This can be developed in line with practice and individual needs as the HCA becomes more confident and integrated within the practice team. To ensure that skill and knowledge levels are maintained, competence must be assessed on a regular basis by a registered practitioner, usually the general practice nurse, with any appropriate training and support put in place as necessary (*see* Chapter 3 on competence).

As the role of the HCA develops, new progression routes are being established. The role of Assistant/Associate Practitioner is one such role, which sits at level 4 of the career framework[12] between an HCA who may or may not hold an NVQ and a qualified registered nurse. Assistant Practitioners do not have professional registration, but are equipped with skills similar to those of a registered nurse. They are involved in delivering protocol-based clinical care that has previously been in the remit of registered health professionals. They take on a higher level of responsibility and run independent clinics under the direction and supervision of a registered health professional, such as a nurse or physiotherapist. This role is well established in radiography, for example, and has helped to develop a career structure for individuals who either want to advance, but do not wish to become registered health professionals, or who wish to gain professional qualifications. It gives the employer the opportunity to look at skills gaps within the team and to decide at what level these should be filled.

The role of the HCA has grown over the years, and they continue to take on a wider range of tasks. There is discussion about whether HCAs should be involved in extended tasks, such as administration of the flu vaccine, and cervical cytology. Each practice will have its own views on what an HCA should or should not be undertaking. However, in the ever changing world of health care the need for each part of the practice team to grow and develop is recognised. The principle for expansion of the HCA role is that they should not be required to make clinical judgements, but are capable of taking on many clinical tasks within defined protocols.

General practice nurses

Although role development can be seen in terms of moving from practice nurse to advanced nurse practitioner or consultant nurse, there are other options available. Where nurses hold a particular interest they could become a Practitioner with Special Interests (PwSI).[26] This role allows for development of a specialist skill to supplement the important generalist role, and encourages delivery of a high-quality specialist service with improved access to meet the needs of a PCT or group of practices.

> 'The services we offer are very patient centred. Our clinics are local, easy to access and give patients the confidence of knowing they can see someone they know has the time to spend with them. We don't diagnose. Our role is to troubleshoot, advise, support and educate.'
> Nurse Practitioner with Special Interests (diabetes)

Another opportunity to develop the role of the nurse in general practice is that of Nurse Partner. The new primary care contracts comprising General Medical Services (nGMS), Personal Medical Services (PMS) and Alternative Provider Medical Services (APMS) support nurses and practice managers who wish to become partners in a general practice.[27] The number of nurse partners is beginning to grow, and the Queen's Nursing Institute has part of its website dedicated to nurse partners,[28] to support those who are consider-ing this option.

The benefits of becoming a nurse partner could include:

- greater autonomy and independence
- the opportunity to bring a different professional perspective to decision making on clinical and business issues within the practice
- a greater degree of job satisfaction
- improved teamwork, with the opportunity to provide an important leadership role for other nurses within the practice
- the opportunity to be involved in the strategic planning of the practice
- profit sharing.

Summary

- As patient-led services continue to grow within primary care, the opportunities for the practice nursing team to develop will also grow.
- Developing the skill mix within the team, and using nurses and HCAs with varying levels of knowledge and expertise, means that the patient will benefit by seeing the right person, in the right place, at the right time, and receive the care that is most appropriate for them.
- The practice will benefit by employing a range of staff with varying levels of skill who are able to provide cost-effective appropriate care.

References

1   www.brightonandhovepct.nhs.uk/healthprofessionals/generalpractice/practicenurs-ing/healthcareassist/index.asp

2   Department of Health. *Our Health, Our Care, Our Say: a new direction for community services.* London: Department of Health; 2006.

3   Mullally S. Extending the nursing role. *Health Technology Assessment Programme, Themed Update.* May 2004.

4   Walsh N, Roe B, Huntington J. Delivering a different kind of primary care? Nurses working in personal medical service pilots. *J Clin Nurs.* 2003; **12:** 333–40.

5   Department of Health. *The NHS Plan: a plan for investment, a plan for reform.* London: Department of Health; 2000.

6   Department of Health. *Modernising Nursing Careers.* London: Department of Health; 2006.

7   Department of Health. *Liberating the Talents: helping primary care trusts and nurses to deliver the NHS Plan.* London: Department of Health; 2002.

8   Department of Health. *Commissioning a Patient-Led NHS.* London: Department of Health; 2005.

9   Royal College of Nursing. *Defining Nursing.* London: Royal College of Nursing; 2003.

10 Wanless D. *Securing Our Future Health: taking a long-term view.* London: Department of Health; 2002.

11 Nursing and Midwifery Council. *Implementation of a Framework for the Standard for Post-Registration Nursing*; www.nmc-uk.org

12 Skills for Health Career Framework; www.skillsforhealth.org.uk/careersframework

13 Department of Health. *Modernising Nursing Careers Review*. CNO Bulletin, December 2005/January 2006. Issue 44; www.dh.gov.uk

14 Working in Partnership Programme; www.wipp.nhs.uk

15 Laurant M, Reeves D, Hermens R *et al*. Substitution of doctors by nurses in primary care. *The Cochrane Database of Systematic Reviews. Issue 4*. Oxford: Update Software; 2005.

16 Keeney S, Hasson F, McKenna H *et al*. Nurses', midwives' and patients' perceptions of trained health care assistants. *J Adv Nurs*. 2005; **50:** 345–55.

17 Wanless, D. *Securing Good Health for the Whole Population: final report*. London: Department of Health; 2004.

18 Gray J. Time to focus on HCAs (editorial). *Nurs Standard*. 2002; **16:** 3.

19 Nursing and Midwifery Council. *Code of Professional Conduct: standards for conduct, performance and ethics*. London: Nursing and Midwifery Council; 2004.

20 Department of Health. *The Regulation of the Non-Medical Healthcare Professions*. London: Department of Health; 2006.

21 Spilsbury K, Meyer J. Making claims on nursing work. Exploring the work of health care assistants and implications for registered nurses' roles. *J Res Nurs*. 2005; **10:** 65–83.

22 Department of Health. *New GMS Contract 2006/2007*. London: Department of Health; 2006.

23 Department of Health. *Practice-Based Commissioning: achieving universal coverage*. London: Department of Health; 2006.

24 Department of Health. *Practice-Based Commissioning: early wins and top tips*. London: Department of Health; 2006.

25 Jenner D. Seven tips to speed up your plans for commissioning. *Doctor*. 2006; **21 March:** 52.

26 Department of Health. *Practitioners With Special Interests: implementing a scheme for nurses with special interests in primary care*. London: Department of Health; 2003.

27 Natpact. *Nurse Partners;* www.natpact.nhs.uk/uploads/2004_Dec/Nurse%20 Partner%20 Factsheet%20FINAL.pdf

28 Queen's Nursing Institute. *Nurse Partners;* www.qni.org.uk/Nursepartners.htm

2

Employment of nurses and health care assistants in general practice

This chapter looks at principles of good employment practice for nurses employed in general practice. It provides ideas and examples of good practice. Awareness of employment issues is raised in order to help to promote favourable terms and conditions and increase job satisfaction.

Contents

Introduction

Nurses working in general practice are members of relatively small organisations, in contrast to other community nurses who are employed by primary care trusts (PCTs). Direct employment by a practice can bring both advantages and disadvantages. Benefits may include more flexibility and opportunities arising from employment within a small business. Conversely, human resource practices may be less rigorous than within large organisations, and this could result in fewer policies for the protection of staff. The principles of employing staff who can provide the best, most effective care for patients are outlined in *A Health Service of all the Talents*.[1] This recognises the importance of maximising the contribution of all staff, including general practice nurses and health care assistants (HCAs), to patient care.

Patient-led services and the drive for quality recognise that staff skills should be developed according to patient need, not professional group. General practitioners (GPs) are the most expensive commodity within a practice, and many Quality Outcome Framework (QOF)[2] points can be gained by organising the primary care team as a whole to ensure that patients receive appropriate care from appropriate individuals. Now that many general practice nurses are learning more advanced clinical skills and increasing their management of long-term conditions, this allows for the development of HCA roles. This development will require initial nursing supervision of less complex tasks in order to create a valuable skill mix within the practice.

The new General Medical Services (nGMS) contract[3] has provided resources to support role development and higher-quality services. It offers practices the opportunity to:

- reconfigure the skills base of the workforce
- improve quality
- manage workloads
- improve the working lives of all staff within the practice.

Identifying good employment practice

The introduction of practice-based commissioning (PBC)[4] offers new opportunities for all staff to expand their knowledge and expertise. General practices with good employment practice will be better placed to recruit and retain high-calibre staff who will help to deliver a greater range and quality of services. The Royal College of Nursing (RCN) has developed an employment charter for practice staff, which lays out the basis for a good employment strategy.[5] This states that practices should:

- follow the spirit and requirements of the relevant national human resource strategy
- provide an up-to-date written contractual statement and job description for every post
- link salaries to national scales, providing annual increases in line with national pay awards
- offer staff a personal training and development plan
- ensure that staff have the right to join and be represented by a trade union of their choice, suffering no disadvantage as a result
- offer health professionals a source of professional advice and support within the PCT
- have written procedures to handle disciplinary matters and grievances, following guidance published by the Advisory, Conciliation and Arbitration Service (ACAS)[6]
- have a written health and safety policy, based on the concept of risk assessment
- observe the requirements of the Working Time Regulations[7]
- have a system for recording accidents and violent incidents involving staff, including verbal or other abuse
- have a written equal opportunities policy and follow good practice in making appointments, staff management, terms and conditions of employment, training opportunities and promotion
- have a written policy on sickness absence, including sick pay arrangements that apply in practice.

By following guidelines such as these, and any new legislation such as the *Employment Equality (Age) Regulations* 2006,[6] practices can ensure that their employment practice is of the highest standard.

This is a dynamic time to be working in general practice as a nurse or an HCA. *The NHS Plan*[8] highlighted the importance of primary care and caring for people in the community. A career in general practice nursing can enable nurses and HCAs to use a broad range of skills, ranging from giving advice on minor illness to caring for patients with serious and debilitating conditions. General practice should provide a flexible and responsive arena that promotes and encourages role development and autonomy for practice nurses and HCAs. However, many nurses working in small practices can suffer from professional isolation. It is therefore particularly important for nurses in general practice to be aware of their employment rights and to be satisfied that they are being treated fairly and appropriately by comparison with other community nurses.

Angela, practice nurse from Stoke-on-Trent

'I love my job as a general practice nurse. Working in general practice means that you get to know patients really well because they come back to see you with different conditions from time to time. You also get to know the whole family, as they're all registered with the practice, and that really makes you feel as if you know them. It's very rewarding to help patients with long-term conditions manage their illness more effectively through patient education and monitoring.'

Anne, health care assistant from Birmingham

'I enjoy working in primary care – it's much nicer than working in a hospital. I can get to know the patients and I get to see them more than once.'

Nurses working in general practice should expect all policies and procedures within the practice to be in line with current employment law. Nurses or HCAs who are hoping to start a career in general practice will want to know the best route to take and how they can be sure of finding the right job for them. The recruitment process should be viewed as an opportunity both for the employer to select the right candidate and for the nurse to select the right job.

Job descriptions and person specifications

Before recruiting a new nurse or HCA, the practice should decide what they need. A *skill mix audit* (*see* Chapter 6, Tool 6.2) is useful for looking at all the jobs in the practice, reviewing who currently does them, and considering whether roles could be redesigned or new roles introduced. A job analysis is also useful for compiling a job description.

---

1   Identify the tasks involved in a job.
2   Look at how, why and when the tasks are performed.
3   Identify the main duties and responsibilities of the job.
4   Consider the physical, social and environmental conditions of the job.

Figure 2.1 Job analysis

A job description that clearly reflects the job's purpose should be created.

These should include the following information.

- **The proposed title of the job.** Practice nurses and HCAs work under a variety of titles (e.g. it is estimated that HCAs have been known by 84 different titles across the NHS 'family'). For consistency it is recommended that job titles are standardised across a PCT.
- **The main purpose of the job.** This should be summarised in one sentence.
- **The objectives of the job.** These clearly identify the activities involved and how they should be carried out.
- **The scope of the job.** This indicates the importance of the job and the degree of responsibility. It should demonstrate who the nurse or HCA is accountable to and, if this is different from the line manager, the way in which this responsibility is allocated.
- **Salary for the post.** Ideally this should be linked to *Agenda for Change* in order to provide parity with NHS colleagues.
- **Training and development.** This should indicate time allocated for training and development.

Figure 2.2 Job descriptions

There should also be a person specification to provide guidance on the essential and desirable personal qualities required for the post.

Person specifications

Tool 2.1 An example of a person specification template

This example provides ideas on how to draw attention to any attributes that may be required for work in general practice.

Title of post:
Grade/band:

Essential attributes:
Requirements necessary for safe and effective performance.

Desirable attributes:
Where available, these elements will contribute to optimal performance.

Qualifications and training:
These would need to be listed.

Knowledge/skills/experience:
This would include any specialised clinical skills relevant to the role.

Personal qualities:
For example, motivation, reliability, commitment to teamworking, and problem-solving and decision-making skills

Requirements due to nature of the working environment:
For example, travel between sites.

The WiPP website (www.wipp.nhs.uk) includes tools relating to the employment of general practice nurses (GPNs) and HCAs, and provides examples of job descriptions. Looking at a range of different job descriptions can help to demonstrate the variety of roles that could be incorporated within a practice. As there is such diversity within general practice nursing, it is important to ensure that any applicants have read the job description carefully, and that it matches individuals' requirements or expectations. For example, some jobs might focus on the management of long-term conditions, whereas others may focus on seeing patients with minor illness requiring same-day advice and treatment. For HCAs, the emphasis may be on single task areas, such as phlebotomy or preparation for minor surgery, or it may have a wider remit, to include screening, new patient checks, administration and health promotion.

Terms and conditions of employment: what to look for

Terms and conditions should be made clear prior to acceptance of a post. Although it may be possible to negotiate some changes before the *contract of employment* is signed (e.g. hours of work, pay and holiday entitlement), these are legally binding once a contract has been signed by both parties. In particular, applicants may want to know:

- whether they are entitled to study leave in order to attend training events
- whether holiday entitlement excludes bank holidays and statutory days
- whether the practice provides NHS pension contributions
- whether any travelling is involved within the role (e.g. domiciliary visits may be required, or visits to nursing homes). If this is the case, there should be clear guidance for remuneration relating to this
- if the practice has a branch surgery, it should be made clear whether nursing staff are required to work at both bases.

All new employees should receive a contract within two months of starting work, and this should be kept in a safe place by the practice and a copy given to the employee. Retaining the contract within a personal development review folder would be appropriate, as it is sometimes useful to refer to the job description when considering an individual's performance over the past year, prior to annual appraisal. Further information and an example of a contract of employment can be found on the ACAS website (www.acas.org.uk).

Practices that are direct employers of nurses and HCAs can determine their own pay levels. The RCN and the nGMS contract encourage practices to employ staff on the terms and conditions of *Agenda for Change*.[9] This revised pay banding system has been successfully adopted by the NHS, but in general practice this remains voluntary.

Agenda for Change (AfC)

This new system relating to pay and conditions of all NHS non-medical staff is based on job evaluation. This means that all staff transferring to this system will need to complete a job-matching process in order to establish their pay banding. Pathways for career development are outlined in the Knowledge and Skills

Framework.[10] The advantages of this system are that the nurse's role will be more clearly defined and there will be financial remuneration for advanced knowledge and skills. AfC terms and conditions are more generous than the previous Whitley Council arrangements – for example, there is more annual leave entitlement.

PCTs will provide advice on how practices can move to *Agenda for Change* principles if they so wish; human resource (HR) departments will have a lot of experience.

It is important to remember that if the practice adopts AfC this applies to all staff, *not just the nursing team.* It may be a worthwhile exercise to calculate the financial impact on the practice prior to discussing the process with staff. For example, introducing the holiday element of AfC will result in extra cover being needed to ensure that there is adequate staffing at all times.

It is not possible for GPs to choose to implement some aspects of AfC but not the package in its entirety. It may be that some staff are disadvantaged by AfC, and the financial impact of this also needs to be considered. If a practice decides to adopt AfC, adequate time and resources should be allocated to the process, as it is important that staff are supported during these changes. It will be helpful if someone acts as project manager during the process.

> For more information about *Agenda for Change*, see *Agenda for Change: NHS Terms and Conditions of Service Handbook,*[11] the *NHS Job Evaluation Handbook*[12] and the information booklet *Agenda for Change: What Will it Mean for You?*[13]

As general practices vary in size from large partnerships in medical centres with 10 or 12 GPs to single-handed practices, so does the number of nurses employed, ranging from a large team of nurses and HCAs to only one nurse. Different working environments suit different people and personalities, so it is important that all aspects of the role and working environment are considered by applicants. Nurses or HCAs expressing interest in a post should be encouraged to make an informal visit to the practice in order to get a feel for the atmosphere and prevailing culture. They should not assume that all general practices will be the same!

Tool 2.2 can be used to consider any advantages and disadvantages of a particular practice. Practice managers may find it useful to complete the same tool to see how their practice might be perceived by others.

Tool 2.2 How attractive is the practice as an employer?

Notes
How important is this to you?
1 = very
2 = quite
3 = not

Image and reputation
Comments from existing staff and patients
A pleasant working environment

Friendly atmosphere
Good socialisation among work colleagues

Training and education opportunities
Induction programme available?
Mentor/assessor available?
Clinical supervision available?
Learning resources available within the practice?
Staff willing to teach in-house?
Protected time for continuing professional development (CPD)?

Employment conditions
Level of pay and benefits – are they linked to *Agenda for Change*?

Good HR practices
Flexible working
Robust contractual agreement
Clearly identified line manager to provide support

Individual performance review
Annual appraisal?
Personal development plan?
Goals and action plans for staff with difficulties?

Promotion and development opportunities
Are there opportunities to progress?
Is career development actively encouraged?
Is CPD supported with funding and protected time?

Communication
Does the practice have regular team meetings involving nurses/HCAs?
Does the practice involve nurses/HCAs in developing strategies?

Applying for a post in general practice nursing

Most PCTs will have a practice nurse lead who is likely to know of current or future vacancies, so anyone looking for a post could be advised to make contact with this person. It is useful for individuals to send in a copy of their curriculum vitae (CV) to practices or the PCT so that their qualifications and experience can be matched up with particular practice needs where possible.

Nursing posts in general practice are successfully advertised in a variety of different forums, including:

- local newspapers
- national nursing press
- the Internet (e.g. NHS jobs (www.jobs.nhs.uk), PCT websites or vacancy bulletins
- Jobcentre Plus (www.jobcentreplus.gov.uk).

Applying for a post as a health care assistant

HCAs are helping general practice to provide more services to their patients by taking on less complex but important tasks that have traditionally been performed by qualified nurses.

By looking at the job description you will be able to see which tasks the practice will expect you to undertake. If tasks are listed that you are not yet competent to perform, you may wish to ask about training.

As an HCA you will want to consider not only the location in which you want to work, but also the role that you will be undertaking. You will want to know basic information such as:

- what the practice is like
- whether a uniform is provided
- whether staff are treated with respect
- whether HR policies and procedures are in place to ensure protection and fairness
- whether there is an opportunity to learn and develop both personally and professionally
- whether there is a space or desk in which to keep personal items
- whether there are facilities for lunch breaks
- whether you can work on a part-time basis or as part of a job share.

Application forms

Application forms should be completed in a way that demonstrates the skills that you can bring to a post. Shortlisting for interview will be based upon the content and quality of the completed application forms, so make sure that you pay attention to detail when completing an application form. Tool 2.3 provides guidance on completing application forms.

Interview

An interview is a two-way process. It is not only an opportunity for the practice to assess what the individual can bring to the job, but also an opportunity for the applicant to see whether they would like to take the job. The HCA toolkit on the WiPP website (www.wipp.nhs.uk) offers hints and tips on how to complete a successful interview.

Mentor support for HCAs

As an HCA you will have tasks delegated to you by a registered nurse who is professionally accountable for ensuring that you are competent to undertake the task. It is essential for you to feel that you have support from the practice nurses with whom you work.

Wherever possible it is helpful for new HCAs to have a designated 'buddy' to work alongside in order to learn the basics. It may also be useful to develop a formal link to a more experienced member of staff who can act as a mentor. The role of mentor is discussed in Chapter 5.

HCAs may occasionally be employed in a practice without a general practice nurse (although this is rare, and not recommended). In this case the practice would need to investigate ways of gaining appropriate support, through either the PCT or a neighbouring practice. Ideas on how you link with general practice nurses or HCAs in other practices are provided in the support information on the HCA WiPP website (www.wipp.nhs.uk/ 43.php).

Richmond and Twickenham PCT HCA Forum

Richmond and Twickenham PCT set up an HCA Forum where HCAs from general practice can meet to talk about their jobs and what happens in different practices. It has given HCAs a voice for putting forward their views on many different topics (e.g. uniforms). HCAs now keep in touch outside of the meetings. They help each other in a variety of ways (e.g. explaining how to use particular pieces of equipment or new patient procedures). The HCA Forum also raises awareness about training and gives the HCAs a point of contact for support, if needed.

Professional support

As an HCA you are not currently required to register with a professional organisation. Joining a union such as UNISON, the RCN or a medical defence organisation, such as the Medical Defence Union (MDU), can provide a wide range of support and information. For example, if you are asked to undertake a task that you have not been trained to do, you could ask a union for advice and guidance which is objective and independent from the practice. For further details contact www.unison.org.uk, www.rcn.org.uk or www.mdu.org.uk.

Review of progress

HCAs should have regular contact with a practice nurse who can provide support in order to build their confidence. Keeping a reflective diary recording your experiences would be a useful way to prompt questions whenever you are reviewing your progress together.

Tool 2.3 provides useful practical advice for nurses and HCAs looking to apply for a post in general practice.

Tool 2.3 How to complete an application form

1 Read the job description and the person specification carefully.
2 Take a photocopy of the blank application form to fill out in rough to start with.
3 Follow any instructions on the form.
4 **Education and qualifications.** Give details of any education, training and qualifications, starting with the most recent. It is important to include all the skills that are relevant to the role. This will include both clinical skills (e.g. experience of helping elderly people with personal hygiene, moving and handling) and non-clinical skills (e.g. reception work, booking appointments, filing, etc.).

5 **References.** You will need to give the names and addresses of two people who will be able to write a reference for you. One of the referees should be your current employer, or your last employer if you are unemployed or not working. If you have never worked it could be a teacher or lecturer. The practice will usually write to your referees if you are invited for interview. If you do not want them to be contacted at this stage, you should make a note of this on the application form.

6 **Employment history.** It is important to show details of the key responsibilities in your current job if you have one, and briefly describe the duties of any previous roles and also the reasons for any breaks in your career (e.g. maternity break).

7 **Further details section.** This section gives you the opportunity to say why you think you are the best person for the job. Use the information on the job description and person specification to explain how your skills and experience match the requirements of the job. Include any experience gained through voluntary work, caring responsibilities or running a home. You can use an additional sheet of paper, but be careful not to make the application too long.

8 Ask a friend to read through your application and make sure it makes sense.

9 Complete the form using **black** ink or ballpoint pen. Write clearly and neatly so that it is easy to read.

10 Once you have completed the form, photocopy it again so that you know what you have put in it. Make sure that you can talk about all the information you have given.

11 Remember to return the application form to the practice by the specified date.

12 If you are invited for interview, remember to phone the practice if the letter asks you to confirm that you will be attending.

Applying for a post as a general practice nurse

General practice provides an ideal setting for nurses to make good use of a variety of skills through contact with a wide range of patients in the community. Successful applications for a post should demonstrate a broad range of skills that will bring clear advantages to the practice. Although application forms may be required in order to provide a standardised approach, it is common practice for nurses to send a CV, which can clearly illustrate an individual's skills and knowledge. Tool 2.4 provides guidance on creating a CV that clearly identifies your assets.

Interview

An interview panel should ideally consist of individuals who are likely to work closely with the practice nurse. This might be the practice manager (for non-clinical duties) and a senior nurse or GP (for clinical matters). A multi-disciplinary panel will ensure a well-considered appointment. Some practices choose to involve patient representatives in the selection process. Those candidates attending for interview who have prepared well in advance will stand out.

- If you have taken the time and trouble to find out about the practice beforehand, this shows that you are highly motivated and it suggests that you have a thorough approach to work. Phone to request an informal visit, or look at the practice website or information leaflet.
- Consider the interview questions you are likely to be asked and rehearse your answers.
- The practice is likely to ask about your future ambitions and strengths and weaknesses, so make sure that you have thought about these in advance. Chapter 5 will help you with this.
- Prepare a range of questions that you can ask the interview panel, as there should be an opportunity for this at the end of the interview. Your questions may include asking whether there will be a formal induction process or if training and development is encouraged as part of ongoing development.
- Don't forget to take your professional portfolio and evidence of your personal identity, qualifications and current NMC registration. However, it is important to be aware that production of an NMC Registration PIN card does *not* constitute proof of professional registration. Employers will need to check this via the NMC free registration confirmation service, which can be accessed at www.nmc-uk.org/aSection.aspx? SectionID=19.
- Any post that is offered will be subject to a Criminal Records Bureau check, occupational health clearance and confirmation of suitability from referees.
- Ask when you will be informed of the results of the interview, and advise the panel of how you would like to be informed (by phone or letter).

Mentor support
Having a mentor (*see* Chapter 5) to provide support and guidance, especially in the early days, will help you to settle into a post more quickly. Although GPs may be happy to act as a 'buddy', support from a fellow general practice nurse who understands the nursing ethos and the NMC *Code of Professional Conduct*[14] will be invaluable. This may be a nurse from within the practice, but if there is no other practice nurse or if other nurses' hours do not coincide with yours, mentorship will need to be provided from outside the practice. The PCT professional lead for practice nursing should be able to provide advice on suitable mentors.

Tool 2.4 Hints and tips on compiling a CV[15]

This tool is useful for nurses who are applying for a job in general practice and who need to be able to demonstrate their strengths in order to secure an interview.

Your CV is your shop window. It has to be good enough to get you that interview so that your undoubted qualities have an opportunity to shine through. Pay attention to the following points.

1 A poorly organised CV may be interpreted as evidence of poor communication skills. Think carefully about layout. Make sure that your strengths are clearly presented.

2 Don't go into too much detail about your earlier years, but make sure that all dates are correct and there are no gaps that you will need to account for. If you have had a career break, be prepared to justify it.

3 Tailor your CV for each application. Identify important information in the advertisement and the person specification, and draw the attention of the people who are shortlisting to your suitability by summarising your key strengths on a front sheet.

4 Consider a competency-based CV. Explain how you are competent for the job for which you have applied. This should not concentrate on the posts you have held, but on what you have achieved within them.

5 Spelling mistakes are inexcusable. Get someone to proofread your CV for you for errors relating to spelling and grammar. Consider asking a senior colleague for their comments.

6 There are many ways in which to structure a CV, and you should consider an initial summary box that describes you and your achievements to date, or a variety of headings that you feel would highlight your strengths effectively.

Starting a new job

Any new starters in general practice will need to demonstrate their competence and capabilities as soon as possible. The NMC *Code of Professional Conduct*[14] states that 'nurses must be aware of and work within their own level of competence to maintain professional standing and patient safety.' This is equally applicable to HCAs, even though they are not bound by a professional code in the same way. Although new employees may want to impress, it is vital for the practice to understand what they are able to do, and what they are not yet able to do without further training or education. A willingness to learn is one of the most important attributes for nurses and HCAs working in general practice.

Legal obligations for employment

Although nurses and HCAs may be employed by relatively small practices, they should be confident that the practice is complying with legal requirements that offer protection to staff. These include the following.

* Personnel records must be kept for all employed staff, including nurses and HCAs. The nurse or HCA has the right to see their own individual records on request.
* Practices should provide a formal period of induction, for which a named member of staff takes responsibility.
* An agreed disciplinary/grievance procedure should be in place that adheres to the Advisory, Conciliation and Arbitration Service (ACAS) code of practice.

- A written procedure manual covering employment policies must be available to staff. This will include policies on equal opportunities, bullying and harassment, maternity leave and sickness absence.
- Nurses and HCAs have the right to join the NHS Superannuation Scheme. It is good practice for the practice to contribute towards this.
- A degree of flexibility in working hours should be offered to allow nurses and HCAs to cope with unexpected family issues.
- The working environment should be safe and comfortable.
- If *Agenda for Change* has been adopted by the practice, the terms and conditions of employment should reflect the principles within this.
- All nurses and HCAs require personal development plans for review at annual appraisal.
- Nurses and HCAs must have access to mandatory training updates on a regular basis.
- IT access should be available to nurses or HCAs during all clinical consultations. It is also preferable that they have access to email (via their own email address), the Internet, Intranet and NHSnet resources.
- GP employers should be aware of the boundaries imposed by the NMC *Code of Professional Conduct*[14] when delegating duties to nurses and HCAs.
- NMC registration for nurses should be checked every year to ensure that it has been updated, as an annual payment is now required.
- Practice nurses must maintain a portfolio of learning as required by the NMC which demonstrates achievement of the minimum standards of 5 days of study leave every 3 years in order to renew annual registration. It would be good practice for HCAs to adopt similar standards.

Professional indemnity

It is strongly recommended that nurses and HCAs are members of a trade union or professional organisation that provides individual professional indemnity.

Vicarious liability for acts and omissions is provided by employers if:

1 the employee was acting in the course of their employment (with regard to time, place, etc.)
2 the employee was doing a job which they are employed to do
3 the employee works within the employer's policies.

Nurses should be aware that if they use their own clinical judgement to deviate from practice guidelines, they cannot rely on vicarious liability provided by the practice, and would therefore need their own indemnity. Each indemnifying organisation has different attractions, so it is worth shopping around to find the most suitable package. Many of these organisations have 24-hour helplines, which can be extremely reassuring if adverse clinical incidents occur and immediate advice is required. It is often the case that the potential gravity of a situation is only appreciated by individuals in the middle of the night!

Induction

A good employer should recognise the importance of induction to the practice, and devise a structured programme to ensure that there are introductions to relevant people, situations and ways of working. New recruits to practice nursing could contact the PCT or local university to find out whether they run an introductory practice nursing course.

Good induction is likely to lead to better retention and to staff who are more settled and secure in their practice. Detailed information relating to induction, which will be particularly helpful to employers or nurses who are asked to set up a programme for a new starter, is available on the WiPP website (www.wipp.nhs.uk).

A comprehensive induction programme for nurses and HCAs will:

- help to define the role and increase confidence and effectiveness
- provide clear guidance as to where the role fits within the general practice team
- promote safe and effective working in a new environment
- encourage commitment to the practice
- quickly dispel the feeling of being new.

When putting together an induction programme, the priorities and goals for the first day, the first week and the first month should be considered. Tool 2.5 provides an example of how this can be done.

Tool 2.5 What to cover in an induction

An induction programme will provide documentary evidence using specific checklists, and a learning plan to demonstrate compliance with QOF standards. A personal record of achievement should also be kept by individuals.

Contents:
Date achieved:

The **first day** could include the following:

- introduction to the immediate practice colleagues
- practical information
- a tour of the surgery
- health and safety (fire exits, fire extinguishers, first-aid kit)
- toilets and hand-washing facilities
- locker and changing facilities
- identity badge and code of dress
- meeting with mentor to identify areas of ability and discuss role and responsibilities.

The **first week** could include the following:

- training in the use of the IT system
- introduction to the wider practice team
- reading of the most important practice policies and clinical protocols
- formal meeting with mentor to identify immediate training needs – this may include witnessed consultations in areas such as cervical screening,

health promotion, asthma care, travel health, childhood immunisations or observation of clinics (depending on individual roles)

- practice leaflet made available to identify range of services currently offered
- an opportunity to discuss working arrangements such as procedure for reporting sickness and requesting annual leave.

The **first month** could include:

- meeting arranged with practice nurse facilitator for the PCT to highlight any forums and study days for nurses in general practice and support available
- ensuring that regular meetings with mentor occur.

Locum staff

Within any practice it is likely that locum staff will be needed at some stage to cover for holidays, sickness or study leave. Practices have a responsibility to check the competence and professional standards of any staff who provide cover, in order to ensure that the practice continues to provide safe and effective care. Locum nurses may be available via PCT bank staff and, as the importance of HCAs increases, it may be viable for PCTs to also add HCAs to their bank staff, so that the practice can be supported when staff are sick or on holiday. If so, they should have a standardised quality assurance system whereby competence is guaranteed. Otherwise the practice will have to take on the necessary checks and ensure that a modified induction programme is in place.

If difficulties occur

It is always better to try to resolve any problems at an early stage. If the practice provides clear guidance to staff (e.g. through procedure manuals and contracts of employment), many problems can be resolved by simply talking things through. If a satisfactory resolution cannot be achieved, the ACAS policies and procedures document the steps to take in order to ensure that the ensuing process is fair and equitable to both parties.

The Employment Act 2002 (Dispute Resolution) Regulations came into force on 1 October 2004. They affect both employers and employees. From October 2004, employers have been required by law to have a discipline and grievance procedure. These regulations cover the disciplinary rules for handling discipline, grievance and appeals (full details can be found at www.acas.org.uk or www.dti.gov.uk/er/resolvingdisputes.htm). This law is designed to encourage employers and employees to discuss problems before resorting to a tribunal, and is a three-step process.

Employment from different perspectives

Employer's perspective

Paying attention to good employment practice is fundamental to improving staff recruitment and retention. A robust and equitable employment policy should be in place within the practice in order to attract and retain the highest calibre of staff to deliver appropriate care for patients. There are many sources of support that can be used to ensure compliance with employment rules and regulations, such as NHS Employers (www.nhsemployers.org), the Advisory, Conciliation and Arbitration Service (ACAS) (www.acas.org.uk) and the Department of Trade and Industry (www.dti.gov.uk). PCTs will also give advice and guidance about HR policies, resources and procedures.

PCT's perspective

Although some PCTs employ nurses and HCAs (particularly for PMS practices), the majority are employed by practices themselves. Although this may mean that PCTs have less contact with practice staff than with PCT employees, the PCT still has responsibility for professional guidance and maintenance of professional standards for practice nurses and the HCAs to whom they have delegated tasks. PCTs may be able to support practices with HR policies or procedures or by examining workforce figures across practices to build up a detailed picture that identifies development needs or gaps in service provision. Some PCTs have established a bank of practice nurses who can provide cover for annual or sick leave or attendance at courses. Liverpool PCT recruits, trains and develops new practice nurses and hires them out to practices. Although this often results in the nurses transferring to direct employment with a practice, the PCT can be assured of the standards that are in place and of overall patient safety.

Education provider's perspective

General practices are independent small businesses that operate within the NHS. Knowledge about employment recruitment and retention varies from practice to practice. Education providers are in a prime position to raise standards by offering education to practices to improve their employment knowledge and skills. Many nurses are keen to gain employment within general practice, but find it difficult because they lack experience. Introductory programmes for working in general practice with a clinical component would be attractive to prospective practice nurses and future employers. This could also be the case for HCAs. General practice will look for education providers who are responsive to the needs of the practice and its staff, and who can be relied upon to produce education and training packages that clearly demonstrate competence on completion.

> **Patient's perspective**
>
> Patients are likely to feel more comfortable in a practice that has clearly defined roles for staff which are explained through leaflets, posters or the practice website. Patients will want to know that the practice has a policy for checking qualifications and completing Criminal Records Bureau (CRB) checks to ensure that staff are qualified and competent to undertake the role.
>
> 'As a patient when I go to the doctor's I think about how my needs are going to be met. I'm not so worried about employment laws at that time but more about whether the people I see are competent enough to provide the services I need and professional enough not to talk about me in a derogatory manner when I have gone. If good employment practices help this to happen then that's great.'

Summary

- The majority of nurses and HCAs in general practice are directly employed by practices. Employment practice can vary, and adopting principles of good employment will be beneficial to both employer and employee.
- A structured approach to recruitment will help to get the right person for the right role, avoiding unnecessary work and expense. It is just as important for a nurse to find the right practice as it is for the practice to find the right nurse.
- Applications for posts in general practice nursing should be well thought out in order to maximise the likelihood of success.

References

1   Department of Health. *A Health Service of All the Talents: developing the NHS workforce.* London: Department of Health; 1999.

2   Quality Outcomes Framework information; www.ic.nhs.uk/services/qof

3   Department of Health. *New GMS Contract 2006/07.* London: Department of Health; 2006.

4   Department of Health. *Making Practice-Based Commissioning a Reality.* London: Department of Health; 2005.

5   Royal College of Nursing. *RCN Nurses Employed by GPs: RCN guidance on good employment practice.* London: Royal College of Nursing; 2005.

6   Advisory, Conciliation and Arbitration Service; www.acas.org.uk

7   Department of Trade and Industry. *Your Guide to Working Time Regulations.* London: Department of Trade and Industry; 2003; www.dti.gov.uk/employment/employment-legislation/employment-guidance/page14232.html

8   Department of Health. *The NHS Plan: a plan for investment, a plan for reform.* London: Department of Health; 2000.

9　Department of Health; www.dh.gov.uk/PolicyAndGuidance/HumanResourcesAnd Training/ModernisingPay/AgendaForChange/fs/en

10　Department of Health. *The NHS Knowledge and Skills Framework (NHS KSF) and the Development Review Process.* London: Department of Health; 2004.

11　Department of Health. *Agenda for Change: NHS terms and conditions of service handbook.* London: Department of Health; 2005.

12　Department of Health. *NHS Job Evaluation Handbook.* 2nd ed. London: Department of Health; 2004.

13　Department of Health. *Agenda for Change: what will it mean for you?* London: Department of Health; 2004.

14　Nursing and Midwifery Council. *Code of Professional Conduct.* London: Nursing and Midwifery Council; 2002.

15　Chambers R, editor. *Career Planning for Everyone in the NHS. The toolkit.* Oxford: Radcliffe Publishing; 2005.

3

Competence of nurses and health care assistants working in general practice

This chapter looks at the importance of being able to prove competence in practice, and what is expected within various roles in general practice nursing. Levels of competence are linked to the NHS Knowledge and Skills Framework and the Quality and Outcomes Framework.

Contents

Introduction

As services move from secondary to primary care, the scope for nurses to gain new knowledge and skills increases. The demands of the new GMS contract[1] for modern primary care services have meant that many practice nurses are expanding their range of skills in order to take on new roles. The development of advanced practice has been supported through national directives on nursing such as *The NHS Plan*,[2] *Making a Difference*[3] and *Liberating the Talents*.[4] This in turn has meant that there is an increasing need for skill mix within general practice. Health care assistants (HCAs) are now undertaking work previously performed by health care professionals in order to meet patient and practice needs.

The change in delivery of services brings with it responsibility for the practice to ensure that patient needs are met by appropriately qualified and trained staff who have been assessed as competent to undertake the role. Individuals also have a responsibility to ensure that they do not work beyond their own level of competence. This may sometimes be difficult in a busy general practice where demands from patients and doctors can be considerable.

Identifying the required competences for a particular role will enable the practice, nurses, HCAs and patients to understand the difference between the nursing roles within a practice, and ensure that everyone is competent to undertake the work required.

Defining competence

Nurses and HCAs work at different levels and all make a unique contribution to care. The importance of identifying the level at which individuals within the practice are working is fundamental to creating an effective and efficient quality service. The complexity of care and the knowledge, ability and skills required will determine who should provide the care.

Benchmarking is a way of defining certain criteria for levels of practice in order to provide a safe, quality service. If nurses and HCAs have clearly identified standards in place that they have to meet, this will equip practices with a safe and effective workforce and will also help to identify training requirements or development needs. The Knowledge and Skills Framework[5] has been introduced to the NHS to help to define levels of practice, so it is useful to adopt this as a basis for determining roles, even if a practice has not yet adopted *Agenda for Change*.[6]

Rating scales can be used to check what level of competence is required at what stage. Benner's 'novice to expert' model[7] is used within nursing to define five levels of practice, ranging from novice to expert. This can be used by individuals to provide a broad overview of the level at which they may be working (*see* Figure 3.1). Self-assessment to identify a place within these levels will encourage self-awareness, and this can then be tested out by asking colleagues whether they agree with their self-rating.

What is competence?

Competence (competences in the plural) is the demonstrable ability and skills required to undertake a particular role or set of activities. Competence is in

---

1 **Novice.** This is the stage in skill acquisition where no background understanding of the situation exists, so that context-free rules and attributes are required for safe entry and performance in the situation (e.g. requires rigid protocols from which to work, and can only work under supervision).
2 **Advanced beginner.** At this level individuals can demonstrate marginally acceptable performance. The advanced beginner has enough background experience to recognise aspects of the situation (e.g. can vary the approach used according to the needs of individual patients, but still requires supervision).
3 **Competent.** This stage in skill acquisition is typified by considerable conscious, deliberate planning. The competent stage is evidenced by an increased level of proficiency (e.g. no longer requires supervision for routine tasks, but is aware of own limits with regard to knowledge and skills, and refers to others appropriately).
4 **Proficient.** The proficient performer perceives situations as wholes rather than in terms of aspects, and their performance is guided by maxims. The proficient performer has an intuitive grasp of the situation based upon a deep background understanding (e.g. experienced in the field of work, able to modify procedures appropriately to match different circumstances, and able to advise others on how to perform tasks).
5 **Expert.** This level is reached when the clinician tests and refines theoretical and practical knowledge in actual clinical situations, so an expert has a deep background understanding of clinical situations based upon many past cases (e.g. very experienced, work has been tested in difficult situations, able to teach others with an understanding of the principles and exceptions in the work).

Figure 3.1 Benner's 'novice to expert' model[7]

effect a standard – for example, 'She is a highly competent ('excellent') phlebotomist' or 'His screening for coronary heart disease is competent ('good').'

Competency (competencies in the plural) is more about what a person brings to a job – that is, the knowledge, skills, abilities and personal characteristics which enable successful performance.

Assessment of competence provides evidence of capability for the individual concerned, for the employer, and for patients. Practice nurses or HCAs should welcome any opportunity that encourages assessment of their level of competence, because it means that they will then be working at an appropriate level, making full use of their skills, but not involved in work for which they are inadequately prepared.

When defining levels of competence, it is important to look at the levels below and above the position in question, as this will help to identify the tasks that can be appropriately delegated to others, as well as clarifying the tasks that can be referred on to more senior colleagues.

Establishing national competences

Skills for Health[8] is the Sector Skills Council for the health care sector. It works with a variety of people, including employers, to ensure that those working in the sector are equipped with the right skills to support the development and delivery of health care services. One of its main roles is to develop National Occupational Standards (NOS) and National Workforce Competences (NWC) for use within the health care sector that link, where appropriate, to key Government agendas and targets, such as the National Service Frameworks[9] and the NHS Knowledge and Skills Framework (NHS KSF)[5] as part of *Agenda for Change*.

The Skills for Health website (www.skillsforhealth.org.uk) provides a database of nationally agreed competences to choose from, with electronic tools to support role development.

Skills for Health describes competences[8] as:

> The descriptors of the performance criteria, knowledge and understanding that is required to undertake work activities. They describe what individuals need to do and to know to carry out the activity, regardless of who performs it.

Why use national competences?

National Occupational Standards can be used by practices as a benchmark to assess a person's competence to undertake a role against a set of national standards.

Within a practice there may be some existing competences and standards that are used locally for assessment. Good practice would be to check these against the national competences to ensure that they align with them.

The benefits to a practice of using the national competences are that they:

- create a common language for describing workforce skills
- ensure a common standard for the delivery of safe patient care
- provide a basis for role profiles and job descriptions
- provide a basis for education and training
- support clinical governance
- develop a clear career framework.

How can national competences be used?

They can be used in a number of ways. For example, they could be:

- clustered together to make individual role profiles or team profiles
- used to develop individual knowledge and skills and improve performance
- used as a basis for education and training
- used as a benchmark to assess competence.

By identifying the specific competences required to undertake the practice nurse or HCA role, and providing appropriate training and assessment, the practice will ensure that they have nurses and HCAs with the relevant knowledge and skills to provide safe, effective care.

Assessing competence

Assessment of competence should be completed with a senior supervisor or mentor as part of ongoing employment and career development for practice nurses and HCAs. It should commence within a basic induction programme and follow on from this as the role expands and as new levels of skills are developed.

Formal courses involving assessment will also provide evidence of competence. However, simply attending a course does not guarantee understanding or learning of a subject, so although courses that do not involve any examination or assessment may seem attractive, it is worth noting that attendance on such courses will not provide proof of competence.

As learning within health care is now recognised as being a lifelong experience, it follows that assessment of competence should also be ongoing. This is particularly important in general practice, where roles are continually changing and expanding.

Assessing performance against competences

There are a number of ways in which performance can be assessed. These include:

- self-assessment
- direct observation
- question-and-answer sessions
- reflective discussions
- peer review
- learning log evidence.

Self-assessment

The Skills for Health website provides an online self-assessment tool to assess performance against each of the competences identified in a role profile. This can then be used as a basis for discussion between a nurse or HCA and their supervisor and/or mentor.

A simple rating scale can be used to identify levels of competence, and this should include dates and levels of experience, such as:

1 = not encountered yet
2 = observed only
3 = performed under supervision
4 = performed independently
5 = considered competent by self and supervisor.

If these levels are applied to all elements within a role, it would be reasonable to expect that there could be targets set for achievement over a 12-month period. Any outstanding competences could be identified at appraisal and completed as part of the continuous learning process.

Associated theoretical knowledge is usually best provided by an accredited course (*see* Chapter 4). Prior knowledge or experience, or learning by other methods, should be recorded in a portfolio (learning log) so that this can be accepted if it is presented in the form of verifiable evidence. Tool 3.1 provides an example of how to assess competence using a rating scale.

Tool 3.1 Assessment template

A template assessment tool to assess a person's performance against a National Occupational Standard/competence

Title of National Occupational Standard/competence:

Performance criteria

1 = not encountered yet
2 = observed only
3 = performed under supervision
4 = performed independently
5 = considered competent by self and supervisor

1
2
3
4
5

Note of learning activity planned to meet the gaps, and date achieved:

You need to:

Activity   Date achieved

1

2

3

4

5

Knowledge and understanding

A = I do not know the knowledge and skills required

B = I know the knowledge and skills required, but I don't have them

C = I know and I am developing the knowledge and skills required

D = I have the knowledge and skills required, but I don't use them

E = I have the knowledge and skills required, and I use them regularly

A

B

C

D

E

Note of learning activity planned to meet the gaps, and date achieved:

You need to:

Activity   Date achieved

1

2

3

4

5

Practice nurse/HCA considered competent by self and mentor/supervisor:

Name of practice nurse/HCA:

Name of mentor/supervisor:

Date:

Date for review:

The outcome of the discussions will be an agreement identifying competences that are being performed to the required standard, as well as areas where there are gaps in knowledge.

Documenting assessment is a critical step in providing evidence of the process. Once the evidence has been documented, it can be used in a number of ways. For example, it can be used to:

- demonstrate competence
- reduce the risk of inappropriate delegation of work
- support the practice in demonstrating that it has met the clinical governance agenda
- support a risk management strategy
- support professional and personal development.

Case study: Proving competence

Gina is moving from the North-East to the Midlands, as her husband's job has been relocated. She has worked in practice nursing for several years and is keen to gain a new position as a practice nurse. Although she has attended for one interview, she has not yet managed to find a job in the new locality.

Feedback from the interview reveals that there was no evidence of any of the higher-level clinical skills that were required for the post. This is a shock to Gina, as she is well respected in the practice, undertakes the full range of practice nurse duties and feels that she has all the skills required for work in general practice. However, she has not undertaken any accredited courses that provide this evidence.

She begins to put together a skills inventory of all the things that she can do, and asks the GP and other team members with whom she works to sign the document to indicate that they are satisfied with her proficiency in the outlined areas.

While undertaking this exercise, Gina recalls that much of her learning has arisen from in-house training that followed a structured programme. She includes this training programme (with dates and comments from her GP, who had acted as mentor) in her portfolio, together with her new skills inventory.

She also remembers that many patients have sent letters of thanks and appreciation, and she includes these as evidence of her empathetic nature and good communication skills.

At Gina's next interview she takes her portfolio with her and she finds that it is much easier to demonstrate the skills that she already possesses. She is successful in gaining a new post, but recognises that the new practice will want to reassess her competence within an induction programme so that they are familiar with her level of knowledge and skills and together they can plan her future learning needs.

Peer review

In addition to self-assessment you may also wish to engage in peer review of your performance. Although this may initially feel a little threatening, it can provide great insight. Asking a colleague to comment on your performance is less intimidating than asking your employer or manager. However, it is important to standardise the process so that feedback is systematic and comprehensive. Consider using a structured format such as Tool 3.2.

Tool 3.2 Using peer review to assess competence

Peer review quite simply involves asking colleagues in your team to comment on each other's performance in order to maintain and improve standards. However, before undertaking peer review, certain ground rules need to be established.

- Talk to your colleagues and check that they are willing to participate.
- Establish whether the comments and review are to be confidential between the two of you, or confidential within the confines of the practice team.
- Devise a form that you are all happy to use for reviewed sessions.
- Make sure that whoever is being reviewed receives a copy of the completed form to retain in their portfolio and to use in appraisals if they so wish.
- If peer review involves observation of your consultation with patients, make sure that the procedure is explained to patients so that they have the option of refusing to participate.
- Make sure that the form you use includes a space for recording both good points and points to improve on.
- Check your self-assessment of performance against the peer review to give you confidence in your self-assessment (e.g. if you thought the consultation went really well and you demonstrated some real skills, is this what your peer reviewer thought too?). If there is a complete mismatch of views, you should ask a senior colleague or your mentor to observe and comment on your performance.
- Summarise the learning points so that you can take actions to improve your performance.

Date of review:
Name and signature of practice nurse/HCA being reviewed:
Name and signature of reviewer:
Nature of session observed (e.g. consultation with patient, specific procedure. etc.):
Consent obtained from patient:

Reviewer's comments:

What was good?
This should include any technical expertise or special skills demonstrated, notes on style, etc.

What was not so good?
This should include anything that appeared less skilled, any distracting mannerisms, etc.

In what ways could performance be improved?
This is an opportunity to highlight ways to improve the less skilled aspects that were observed.

Overall comment on performance
This is a general statement that encapsulates the overall standard.

Comments of practice nurse/HCA being reviewed:

Self-assessment of performance
This should be your own appraisal of the situation reviewed, which you should think about and note down before you see your reviewer's comments.

Observations on reviewer's comments
These record whether you think that the reviewer has made a fair assessment and whether you have learned any useful tips or gained insight from the experience.

Action plan resulting from review
This should demonstrate what you have learned from the review and show how you are going to use that learning to improve practice.

Competence from the practice nurse's perspective

The NMC *Code of Professional Conduct*[10] emphasises that nurses must not work beyond their level of competence:

> To practise competently you must possess the knowledge, skills and abilities required for lawful, safe and effective practice without direct supervision. You must acknowledge the limits of your professional competence and only undertake practice and accept responsibilities for those activities in which you are competent.
>
> (Clause 6.2, NMC *Code of Professional Conduct*, 2002)

This means that you need to regularly self-assess your skills. This should be done formally, at least once a year, in your annual appraisal, and any training and education that you need should be recorded in your personal development plan.

If you have a mentor, it will also be useful to discuss your self-assessment with them. You can then draw up an action plan of how you will acquire the knowledge and skills that you require to add to your existing expertise.

If you are undertaking formal education relating to your role, your mentor will probably be required to assess and record your clinical competences. Make sure that you keep any such records within your professional portfolio, as these could be of great value in demonstrating your abilities to any future employers.

The Quality and Outcomes Framework[11] provides new opportunities for general practice nurses to work in more depth with patients who have long-term conditions – taking responsibility for managing and providing their care. This means that new levels of knowledge and skill must be acquired in order to be fully competent.

Competence from the HCA perspective

It is important for you, your patients, the qualified nurses with whom you work and your employers to know that you are competent and able to carry out your assigned duties and any additional tasks that are delegated to you. Therefore you should not feel threatened by anyone wanting to observe your performance, but understand that it is a reasonable requirement for a role that places you in direct contact with patients. If you are ever in any doubt as to whether you can undertake a task proficiently, it probably means that you can't, and you should always discuss this with a qualified member of staff.

If your practice supports you in undertaking National Vocational Qualifications (NVQs), competences will also be assessed by an accredited NVQ assessor. This could be either your mentor/supervisor or an external assessor.

Delegation, accountability and responsibility

The NMC *Code of Professional Conduct*[10] recognises that registered nurses are not the only people who deliver health care.
It states that nurses:

> … may be expected to delegate care delivery to others who are not registered nurses or midwives. Such delegation must not compromise existing care, but must be directed to meeting the needs and serving the interests of patients and clients. You remain accountable for the appropriateness of the delegation, for ensuring that the person who does the work is able to do it and that adequate supervision or support is provided.

Patients need to know who is providing the care, as it is sometimes difficult to differentiate between registered nurses and HCAs.

Delegation

The key to appropriate delegation is the right skill mix for the particular clinical setting, high-quality supervision and adequate preparation in the form of knowledge, skill and competence.

Over time the boundaries of a role can become blurred, and it is very easy for expectations to be placed on roles that go well beyond existing job descriptions and assessed competences. Regular assessments and appraisals will help to identify any issues that can then be addressed.

Accountability

HCAs do not have professional registration. Therefore a practice nurse or registered health professional who supervises the HCA is accountable for the appropriateness of the clinical tasks that are delegated to them. However, HCAs are accountable to the patient for any errors they make through civil law, and are accountable to their employer through their contract.

Legal accountability relates to the obligation of citizens, including nurses and HCAs, to obey the laws of the country and to be able to defend their actions through the court if required to do so. Legal responsibility encompasses civil law (e.g. the duty of care), criminal law (the duty towards to the public) and employment law (the duty to the employer).

Professional accountability relates to the additional obligation of the professions not to abuse trust, and to be able to justify professional actions even when they are not against the law.

In order to achieve accountability, the elements of competence, responsibility and authority need to be considered and understood. For an HCA, *competence* is what a supervisor or assessor assesses, *responsibility* is the inclusion of that task or activity in the job description, and the *authority* to undertake the task or activity is delegated by the registered nurse or other health professional.

The United Kingdom Central Council for Nursing, Midwifery and Health Visiting (UKCC)[12] identified a number of key points regarding the role of HCAs.[13]

- HCAs must work under the direction and supervision of registered practitioners.
- Nurses remain accountable for assessment, planning and standards of care, and for determining the activity of their support staff.
- HCAs must not be allowed to work beyond their level of competence.
- HCAs should be integral members of the caring team.
- HCAs should be encouraged to gain vocational qualifications.
- Nurses should be involved in these developments so that support roles can be designed to ensure that professional skills are used appropriately for the benefit of patients.[6]

Developing rigorous processes for education, training and development and the assessment of competence against national standards will support the appropriate delegation of tasks to HCAs.

- A practice will want to be sure that they have in place systems and procedures to comply with Government legislation and medical defence organisation requirements related to delegation.
- Registered nurses will want to be sure that the person to whom they delegate the task has the knowledge, skills and competence to undertake the delegated work.
- HCAs will want to be sure that they have received the training and support necessary to develop the requisite knowledge and skills, and have been assessed as competent to undertake the task.

There are times when you may be asked to work outside these boundaries, and it is often difficult to refuse to perform a task when asked. Protocols and guidelines for team members help to formulate who does what and when, making the lines of responsibility clear. However, if you are being asked to act outside your role or competences, it might be worth speaking to your line manager or asking if you could discuss your role in more detail at a team meeting.

You may like to look in the HCA Toolkit on the WiPP website (www.wipp.nhs.uk) for ideas on how to say 'No' if you are experiencing difficulties in your practice.

Figure 3.2 Delegation of tasks: what HCAs need to know

> **Example**
> Patsy is a health care assistant working in the asthma clinic with the practice nurse. She measures the peak flow change in a patient who is being assessed for reversibility, having been previously assessed as competent to carry this out following training and education (assessed competence). The role forms part of her job description (responsibility). The practice nurse has delegated this activity (authority) to her in full knowledge of her competence and job description, but retains the professional responsibility, as Patsy does not at present have the backing of a professional body to regulate her accountability.

The WiPP booklet on accountability and delegation[14] gives more specific guidance and can be downloaded from the WiPP website (www.wipp.nhs.uk).

Linking competence with the Knowledge and Skills Framework[5]

The NHS Knowledge and Skills Framework (NHS KSF) has been introduced to help to define levels of practice within the NHS. It is helpful to use this as a basis for determining roles, even where practices have not yet adopted *Agenda for Change*.[6]

Linking competences to the NHS KSF is one way of ensuring that a role is in line with others across the country. The NHS KSF represents the first attempt to relate health care activity and skills to a standardised level.

The NHS KSF consists of 30 dimensions which identify broad functions that are required by the NHS to enable it to provide a good-quality service to the public. Each dimension has four levels which have indicators attached to them, linked to the National Occupational Standards, and which describe how the knowledge and skills are applied at each level.

Job descriptions and competency frameworks for nurses and HCAs linked to the NHS KSF can be found on the WiPP website (www.wipp.nhs.uk). More information on using the NHS KSF can be found at www.rcn.org.uk/publications/ pdf/NHS%20knowledge%20and%20skills%20framework.pdf

The Scottish Framework for Nursing in General Practice[15] also provides a model that identifies components of the roles of staff nurse, specialist practice nurse and advanced practitioner.

Advanced nursing practice

A recent consultation from the NMC has supported the proposal to introduce an additional level of registration for advanced nurse practitioners. This still requires changes to legislation before it can be implemented. This additional sub-part of the nursing register has defined standards for advanced practice. Practice nurses who are currently acting in advanced roles (or using the title 'nurse practitioner') will have the opportunity to prove achievement of these standards. The standards are linked to competence in assessment and treatment, and must be achieved at a minimum of honours degree level.

Advanced practice is different from *specialist practice*, which is an additional qualification approved by the NMC. This qualification has pathways for all branches of community nursing, including practice nursing, but does not necessarily include advanced-level clinical skills.

Competence for nurses and HCAs in general practice from different perspectives

Employers' perspective

The competence required for varying roles within general practice nursing should be clearly defined in order to minimise patient risk. Benchmark standards can be introduced, and mapping competence against these standards will also help to identify any learning needs. The NHS Knowledge and Skills Framework[5] provides a model for distinguishing the requirements for particular posts, and use of this will also facilitate the adoption of *Agenda for Change*. Assessment of competence is essential for delegation of duties within the Quality and Outcomes Framework,[12] and consideration should be given within the practice as to how competence can be measured and monitored.

Strategic perspective

PCTs have a responsibility to ensure that all patient services are delivered in an appropriate manner by suitably qualified staff. This means that they must be confident in the competence of their independent contractors (including GPs and nurses who work in general practice). PCTs may wish to encourage general practices to use the National Occupational Standards to assess standards of practice. Encouraging practices to match competences against the NHS Knowledge and Skills Framework will have the distinct advantage of improving the alliance between nurses in general practice and the rest of the community nursing workforce. PCTs should also ensure that they have assessed the competence of any locum practice nurses; investing in bank staff may facilitate this.

Patient's perspective

Patients should be able to assume that any nurse working in general practice is adequately prepared and competent to undertake the care that they deliver. Practice leaflets should provide some detail relating to the qualifications of nurses. In addition, patients have the reassurance that registration with the NMC for registered nurses is designed to provide some public protection. Patients need to understand that there are varying roles within general practice nursing, all of which demand different levels of skills. Information relating to the different roles could be provided within the practice to provide clarity and reduce unrealistic expectations.

> **Educationalist's perspective**
>
> Educationalists need to be conscious of linking assessment of learning to competence in practice in order to create attractive learning packages that will be welcomed by practice nurses, HCAs and employers alike. Education providers need to stay in touch with the growing demands of clinical practice. The link between NVQs and the National Occupational Standards provides ideal opportunities for HCAs to prove their competence if assessment against these national competences is taken on board within general practice.

Summary

- Defining the competences that are required for a role is a way of identifying whether the practice nurse or HCA has the knowledge, skill or capacity to undertake a particular job or activity.
- Professional registration with the NMC for registered nurses provides evidence of defined standards in terms of clinical practice. At present, HCAs are not subject to professional registration and are therefore not professionally accountable, although they are legally accountable for their actions. This means that nurses who are delegating tasks need to ensure that the person to whom they delegate has the knowledge and skills required to undertake the task and has been assessed as competent by a responsible registered professional.
- Different levels and types of nursing care and skills are required in general practice, and these need to be differentiated so that they are valued and supported at an appropriate level. A nationally defined set of standards provides a benchmark for comparing skills.
- Proven competence is important for clinical governance, as it significantly reduces risk.

References

1 Department of Health. *Investing in General Practice: the new General Medical Services contract.* London: Department of Health; 2006.

2 Department of Health. *The NHS Plan: a plan for investment, a plan for reform.* London: Department of Health; 2000.

3 Department of Health. *Making a Difference: strengthening the nursing midwifery and health visiting contribution to health and healthcare.* London: Department of Health; 1999.

4 Department of Health. *Liberating the Talents: helping primary care trusts and nurses to deliver the NHS Plan.* London: Department of Health; 2002.

5 Department of Health. *The NHS Knowledge and Skills Framework.* London: Department of Health; 2004.

6 Department of Health. *Agenda for Change.* London: Department of Health; 2004.

7 Benner P. *From Novice to Expert: excellence and power in clinical nursing practice.* Menlo Park, California: Addison-Wesley; 1984.

8 Skills for Health; www.skillsforhealth.org.uk

9 National Service Framework; www.dh.gov.uk/PolicyAndGuidance/HealthAndSocial CareTopics/HealthAndSocialCareArticle/fs/en?CONTENT_ID=4070951&chk=W3ar/W

10 Nursing and Midwifery Council (NMC). *Code of Professional Conduct.* London: NMC; 2002.

11 Quality Outcomes Framework; www.dh.gov.uk/PolicyAndGuidance/Organisation Policy/PrimaryCare/PrimaryCareContracting/QOF/fs/en

12 United Kingdom Central Council for Nursing, Midwifery and Health Visiting (UKCC). *Perceptions of the Scope of Professional Practice.* London: UKCC; 1992.

13 Storey L. Delegation to health care assistants. *Pract Nurs.* 2005; **16:** 294–6.

14 Working in Partnership Programme. *Accountability and Delegation.* www.wipp.nhs.uk

15 Scottish Health Executive. *The Scottish Framework for Nursing in General Practice.* Edinburgh: Scottish Health Executive; 2004; www.scotland.gov.uk/Publications/ 2004/09/19966/43291

4

Education and training for nurses and health care assistants in general practice

This chapter looks at the importance of education and training and advises on appropriate approaches to learning, with specific advice for both nurses and HCAs.

Introduction

The terms 'education' and 'training' are often used together, and it is useful to appreciate the differences between them. Education is defined as 'the act of imparting knowledge or skills, or the act of obtaining such knowledge or skills'. Training is defined as 'making proficient', or as 'guiding someone in a particular direction'.

Whereas education may be wide, training is usually focused on specific skills and the knowledge required for those skills to be practised in a competent manner. Useful working definitions are as follows.[1]

- Education is about doing things better.
- Training is about taking on new tasks.

Providing access to training and education opportunities often makes people feel more valued, and as a result they are more likely to remain with an employer. Trained staff add flexibility to the practice team and enable the practice to safely expand its services to meet the needs of the local population. Only someone who is fully trained and assessed as competent can deliver the correct care and minimise risk of harm to patients.

Education and training should not occur as a one-off event. Working within health care involves a process of lifelong learning, and GPNs and HCAs should recognise the need to gain both academic and vocational knowledge and skills to help improve patient care.

Anxieties about learning

Many nurses and HCAs may feel anxious at the prospect of undertaking courses or attending study days. For those who have not studied for some time it is inevitable that there will be feelings of apprehension. The return to formal learning can be quite intimidating. There could be concerns about being able to cope, or memories of unhappy schooldays.

However, adult learning is very different. Most people learn best through experiential learning – that is, learning through doing rather than just listening. This also involves learning through reflecting on practice. Previous experience plays an important role because it provides a building block on which new knowledge and skills can be developed. Formal learning usually includes assessment. This has the advantage of providing reassurance to both individuals and employers that a recognised standard of knowledge and competence has been achieved. For those who are nervous about studying, it will be helpful to talk to colleagues who have undertaken recent study. This will provide an opportunity to discuss expectations and different ways of coping with work and study. Most people are very keen to support personal and professional development, and colleagues often help by providing relevant articles or books that may be useful if they know someone is studying a particular topic area (e.g. diabetes).

Nurses and HCAs who have undertaken significant further training and are taking on increased responsibilities may be considered for re-grading on the salary scale, especially if they are working independently to run nurse-led services.

Education for HCAs

In 1988, the United Kingdom Central Council for Nursing, Midwifery and Health Visiting (UKCC)[2] saw HCAs as taking on the role of housekeeping, clerical work and maintenance of the workplace for health professionals. How things have changed! Now, HCAs are involved in direct patient care, and require defined standards of education and training to ensure competence.

Professional staff who delegate tasks to an HCA need to be confident in the abilities of that individual to perform the tasks in a competent manner. Undertaking a recognised training programme will enhance the HCA's skills, knowledge and attitudes. Programmes that include assessment will also demonstrate practical application of these skills and will reassure the HCA, the practice and patients that any delegated tasks can be undertaken safely.

Within general practice, HCAs are required to work in situations where constant close supervision is not always possible. This means that HCAs need to be able to share in the responsibility for working safely and correctly. Education, training and assessment will help to give them the confidence to do this successfully.

Education for general practice nurses

At present there is no statutory post-registration qualification for practice nursing, although it covers a very broad range of skills and knowledge. Practice nurses come into contact with a wide range of patients, from the very young to the very old and the healthy to the acutely ill. This means that the underlying education required to undertake the role is vast, and relies strongly on the principles of lifelong learning which are supported by the Nursing and Midwifery Council.

Liberating the Talents[3] highlighted the need for flexibility across professional boundaries, and outlined a new framework for nursing in primary care, based on three core functions:

- first contact/acute assessment, diagnosis, care, treatment and referral
- continuing care, rehabilitation and chronic disease management
- public health/health protection and promotion.

Education for all community nurses, including district nurses and health visitors, should therefore have a common core. It is clear from various national policies that nurses in primary care will increasingly take on roles that were previously considered to be the province of the GP. Education and training are important in developing skills to meet these challenges.

All registered nurses are required to keep a portfolio of learning and practice to demonstrate continued professional development (CPD) by achieving the NMC Post-Registration Education and Practice Standards (PREP).[4]

To remain on the professional nursing register, nurses must demonstrate that they meet the standards relating to practice and CPD.

- Practice standard – nurses must work a minimum of 450 hours in practice or undertake an approved 'Return to practice' course within a 3-year period prior to re-registration.
- CPD standard – nurses must take and record CPD within the same 3-year period. The minimum is five days (35 hours) of learning activity relative to their area of practice.

In addition, nurses must keep a personal professional profile of learning activity. Any mandatory training is additional to these requirements. CPD can be accessed in a variety of ways, and employers have a duty to facilitate this.

There is no approved set format for learning, but it must be relevant to the role in which individuals are working.

Ways of learning

Learning occurs in both formal and informal ways. Most learning probably occurs in informal situations, through observing others, talking to others, practising activities, trial and error, or simply working with people 'in the know.'

Informal learning can be recorded in a diary or learning log to provide evidence of transferable skills. Informal learning can also include support groups where individuals can meet and exchange ideas, look at problems and help each other to do the job better.

Formal learning consists of activities such as training courses or workshops, but it is not only what has been learned from these forums but how it translates into practice that makes learning meaningful.

Observation of how others perform tasks and interact with people is a good way of learning. It is most effective when combined with reflection. Observation of individuals with feedback from mentors is another useful way of gaining insight into performance. Time for reflecting and thinking about learning should be built into any supervised activity.

Learning from patients is a constant activity for anyone engaged in practice. This type of learning can be captured, at least occasionally, by recording it in a diary or learning log. Sometimes patients provide direct information from their own knowledge. At other times the questions that patients ask stimulate practitioners to find out information or develop a new skill.

Learning in groups is a common way of approaching learning, and can be valuable. The problems never look that difficult when the solutions are developed in a group with team members, tutors or facilitators. However, finding solutions to a problem when alone can be more difficult for individuals who have relied on other group members to do the thinking for them. Therefore group work should not be relied upon to provide all the answers.

Inter-professional learning enables cross-fertilisation of ideas. Everyone approaches complex problems differently, so working within a team allows individuals to see different aspects of a problem that they might not otherwise consider. This is why inter-professional learning can be so valuable.

Case study: Sadia, practice nurse

'Our practice participates in group learning on a monthly basis. We all get together and talk about a particular clinical topic, such as asthma. Sometimes the practice manager arranges for an outside speaker to attend. It is really interesting to hear about different people's experiences of managing patients with that condition. The doctors often know more about the medication and they are sometimes surprised by the emphasis that practice nurses put on preventive care, and how HCAs can spend considerable time teaching practical skills, such as inhaler techniques. It makes you realise how important everybody's contribution is to improving standards of patient care.'

Support groups can be set up to provide a network for HCAs and/or nurses to share good practice and identify further training requirements. Outside speakers are often invited if a common educational need is identified.

PCT support – some PCTs or practices actively facilitate learning opportunities, and contacting the PCT to see what is available locally or suggest ideas is a good place to start.

Learning through reflection

Much learning will take place during the normal course of work in the practice. It is useful to keep a journal or log to record this learning, both to check that subjects are covered and to help with a learning needs assessment. The purpose of a learning log is to pick out the most personally significant experiences on a particular day and record what has been learned from those experiences. This will involve reflecting on:

- what was most significant
- why this was personally significant
- what has been learned
- any actions that have been proposed as a result.

Reflection can be undertaken in many different ways. Tool 4.1 may be helpful.

Tool 4.1 Example of a reflective practice tool

Fill in each column with memorable patient encounters or issues that you come across in your work. Nurses undertaking this activity could include this in their personal professional portfolio as proof of learning in practice.

Remember always to code your patients' names when using any information that may be seen by others, so that the patients remain anonymous. (For nurses this requirement is noted within the NMC *Code of Professional Conduct*.)

Date:

Patient or problem:

Issue/what happened:

Ideas for learning/what you have learned:

Action plan/what you are going to do about it:

For example:

31 January 2006

Mrs J

Unable to use inhaler device. Patient cannot remember what was shown to her.

This patient needs to have continual reinforcement and education in the use of an inhaler.

Make sure that her inhaler technique is checked on every clinic visit. Set up a prompt to appear on the computer screen to alert staff to this fact.

Learning through reflective practice is about learning from experience. It is viewed as an important strategy for health care professionals and a component of lifelong learning. The act of reflection is seen as a way of promoting the development of autonomous, qualified and self-directed professionals. Although it has been traditionally geared towards registered professionals, it can be an equally rewarding experience for HCAs. Engaging in reflective practice is associated with an improvement in the quality of care, stimulating personal and professional growth and closing the gap between theory and practice.

It is often helpful to use a defined model of reflection, and examples of these can be found in the GPN and HCA Toolkits on the WiPP website (www.wipp.nhs.uk).

Identifying learning needs

Anyone starting a new role is likely to feel overwhelmed, and an induction programme is a good way of identifying any skills and knowledge that need to be developed. However, identifying learning needs and opportunities should be an ongoing process, as these will change over time but they never go away!

A learning and development plan will help both staff and employer to plan what education or training is needed for the role both now and in the future. Nurses and HCAs should consider the following points:

- the amount of time available to commit to study, taking into account personal and work circumstances
- how a personal development plan (PDP) will contribute to the wider practice-based planned clinical governance programme
- the PCT's local delivery plan together with the practice business plan, to see how targets and priorities can be met
- balancing personal learning needs with the needs of the practice. It is vital that educational programmes and CPD fit in with the long-term aims of the practice.

Case study

In her appraisal, Mary identified the fact that she would like to go on a diabetes course. Jane, the other practice nurse, had recently completed one such course at the local university and said it was really good. However, when Mary discussed this with the practice manager she realised that the practice now had the necessary skills to develop a diabetes clinic, and that it would be much more useful for the patients if she attended an asthma course, as no one in the practice had the appropriate expertise to run a clinic, and asthma was known to be a common problem in their local area. Mary was disappointed, but she could see the benefits to the practice of developing her knowledge of asthma. However, she did ask if her interest in diabetes could be noted in case the nurse-led service for diabetes expanded further in the future.

Undertaking a learning needs assessment

A learning needs assessment will help to focus on what is needed for an individual to be more effective in a particular role. This will prevent people undertaking courses that are not particularly helpful, and will avoid any missed learning opportunities. Tool 4.2 can be used by HCAs and nurses to ensure that they gain maximum benefit from CPD.

Tool 4.2 Learning needs assessment[5]

Stage 1: Making your overall learning plan

Here you need to be completely honest with yourself.

1 Identify areas where you need to develop your knowledge, skills or attitudes.
2 Specify topics for learning as a result of changes in your role, responsibilities or organisation.
3 Link into the learning needs of other individuals in your practice.
4 Tie in with the service development priorities of your practice, the PCT or the NHS as a whole.
5 Describe how you identified your learning needs.
6 Prioritise and set your learning needs and associated goals.
7 Justify your selection of learning goals.
8 Describe how you will achieve your goals and over what time period.
9 Describe how you will evaluate your learning outcomes.

The more time you invest in making your plan, the more likely it is that you will focus your learning effectively.

Your PDP will evaluate your progress so far and what your future needs are. Your learning plan is essential for your PDP to take place.

Organising evidence

You should organise all the evidence for your learning into a portfolio:

• for nurses – to provide evidence of CPD as stated by the NMC in the PREP document.
• for HCAs – can be used as evidence for CPD or NVQs.

This evidence of continuing professional development can also be used for job interviews in the future.

It is up to you how you keep this record of your learning up to date, but some examples include either a learning log or a simple A4 file with plastic wallets in which to build up a systematic record of your educational activities.

Stage 2: Using a range of methods to identify your learning needs

Where are you now? What are your roles and responsibilities? What do you need to know? What knowledge, skills and attitudes do you need?

- Your learning needs will encompass the context in which you work as well as your knowledge and skills in relation to any particular role or responsibility of your current post.
- The extent of the learning that you need to undertake will depend on your level of responsibility for a particular role or task – whether you are personally responsible, delegating or contributing.
- Your learning needs will be different if you work in an inner-city practice compared with a rural practice, or if your practice population has a high proportion of minority groups such as immigrants, the homeless or people with special needs.

Your learning should take into account your aspirations for the future in terms of personal or career development, or improvements in the way you deliver care in your practice. Use several different methods to identify your learning needs, as no one method will give you reliable information about all the gaps in your knowledge, skills or attitudes.

You could determine what it is you don't know by:

- asking patients, users and non-users of your service
- comparing your performance against best practice
- comparing your performance against objectives in business plans or national directives
- asking colleagues from different disciplines about ways in which you could improve the ways in which you work with them.

Stage 3: Deciding where you want to go next

Think of it as a journey to another airport. You know that you are at a major airport. You can go in almost any direction and as far as you like. You may need to change planes, or even the type of transport, but you will only reach the desired destination if you have a plan. If you travel without an aim you will probably end up in the wrong place, or even back where you started.

Look back at your aspirations that you set in Stage 2. Each of these is your target destination. You now have to decide the route and how to get there. Changing performance and improving quality can be difficult, and education is the key to this. Initial enthusiasm can soon evaporate in the daily chores of work. Computer-generated reminders or even notes in a diary are helpful to keep you going.

Stage 4: Setting priorities for what and how you learn

Some of the needs in your learning plan will be appropriate for the present circumstances, some will be too costly and others will be too time consuming. Go through again and select those that have clear aims and objectives and that are achievable within the time and money constraints under which you are working. Then rank them in order of priority. You need to set a time limit for achieving these objectives.

Learning styles

People learn in different ways, and using a variety of approaches to acquire new information or skills helps to utilise study time with maximum efficiency.

Tool 4.3 will help to identify the dominant learning style for individuals and to decide on the best ways of learning for them. Using as many different learning methods as possible will help to reinforce learning.

Tool 4.3 Identifying your learning style and ways you can approach learning

Learning styles (adapted from many sources)

Read the word in the left-hand column and then choose which column contains the most answers that suit you. This will be your dominant style of learning.

	Visual	*Auditory*	*Action*
When you cannot spell a word, do you:	Try to visualise the word	Sound out the word	Write down the word to see if it feels right
When talking, do you use words like:	See, picture, image	Hear, tune, think	Feel, touch, hold
Are you distracted by:	Looking at your surroundings or by untidiness	Sounds and noises	Activity and movement
Do you prefer to contact people:	Face to face or in writing	By telephone	While walking or participating in an activity
Do you remember people best when you recall:	Where you met or what they were wearing	What you talked about	What you were doing
When reading, do you prefer:	Descriptive scenes or to imagine the scene	Dialogue or plays	Lots of action, doing things rather than reading
When you do something new at work, do you prefer to have:	A demonstration or see it written on a poster or diagram	Verbal instructions or talk it through with someone	The opportunity to try it out yourself
When you are assembling something, do you prefer to:	Look at the directions and pictures	Have someone read out the directions	Just put it together, and only use the directions if you get stuck
If you need help with a computer program, do you:	Look for pictures or diagrams	Phone a helpline or ask someone	Keep trying different approaches

Honey and Mumford[6] have developed a learning style questionnaire that you can complete yourself to help you to identify your main styles of learning. They identify four different learning styles, and understanding your own approach will help you to identify how you might learn most effectively.

It may be helpful to look at other ways of exploring learning. Tool 4.4 will help you to achieve this.

Tool 4.4 Exploring learning from different angles

Making use of variety when acquiring new information or skills helps you to utilise your time with maximum efficiency.

Try looking at the material in different ways.

• Describe the material out loud, or use a question-and-answer format.
• Use a flowchart or diagram for the material.
• Make an image or a model of the material.
• Play background music as you learn or sing important points out loud.
• Teach someone else.
• Reflect on the material.
• Use index cards with important points arranged in different ways.

Create bite-sized chunks.
If you feel overwhelmed by a particular task, try breaking it down into smaller sections.

Look at the bigger picture.
Sometimes it is good to draw back from a problem and see how it fits into the bigger picture.

Put things into a framework.
Using a structure (e.g. a list) can help you to connect the new materials to things you already know. This reduces the amount you have to learn at one time and increases your confidence that the learning is really working.

Reinforce learning.
You could do this by:

• teaching someone else
• writing about new information.

Demonstrating new skills by teaching someone else can help to reinforce your learning and confidence.

Selecting a course

When you are considering a course, Tool 4.5 will help to identify the kind of questions to ask to ensure that the course really is what is required.

Tool 4.5 Questions to ask about courses

Contact the course provider and find out about what is provided. Ask questions about the following.

1 What the course involves.
- Teaching methods (e.g. workshops, e-learning, videos, etc.).
- Course outline and options.
- Exams and assessment.
- A mixture of teaching and practical work.
- Arrangements for the practical work.
- How much time will it take away from the service provision at work?
- How much work will have to be done at home?

2 What the facilities are like.
- Library and computer availability.
- Will you need a computer at home?
- Refreshments and other provisions for comfort.
- Is the journey reasonable and practical? Is there adequate car parking?
- Are the contact details easy to find and is the training provider responsive to enquiries?

3 Whether there is there any additional support for students.
- Is there a regular system for individual learning?
- Will you need to set aside time for reflection and learning at work?
- Is additional learning support available for special needs (e.g. dyslexia)?

4 How this education provider performs.
- What percentage of students complete their studies?
- Is the information on pass rates and drop-out rates readily available?
- Does the education provider ask for and act on feedback?
- Are its standards checked by an external moderator?

5 What you can do with the qualification.
- Can you progress to other courses (e.g. do Credit Accumulation Transfer Scheme (CATS) and Accreditation of Prior Learning (APL) apply)?
- Is the qualification transferable to other areas of work or other areas of the country?

6 How the course will change your practice.
- What will you be able to do differently as a result of attending the course?

7 How much it will cost.
- Is it affordable for the HCA/general practice nurse/practice/PCT?
- Is any financial assistance available?

Evaluation of learning and professional development

It is good practice to evaluate learning and professional development. Keeping a record of what has been achieved and reflecting on this will help to demonstrate competence to undertake a specific task or role and fitness for purpose.

In addition, if the practice adopts *Agenda for Change* (*see* Chapter 2) and the NHS Knowledge and Skills Framework, it will be easier to demonstrate that the requirements for each of the dimensions have been met over the past 12 months.

After a learning session, Tool 4.6 can be used to review what has been gained. This can be printed off and kept in a portfolio of learning. The tool identifies what worked, what did not work and what would be done differently next time.

Tool 4.6 What have I gained from my learning experience?

See the examples provided below as a guide to how to complete this table. This could be kept as part of your personal portfolio, as a reminder of the learning mechanism that you find most effective for getting maximum benefit from a learning event or session.

Learning experience:

Date and location:

What worked well:

What did not work:

What will I do differently next time?

Example 1:

Spirometry course

1 January 2005
Happy Hospital

Made lots of notes in the session.
Had a chance to ask questions.

Sat at the back, so quite difficult to hear and see at times. I should have looked at my notes after the session to ensure that they would make sense later on.

Sit nearer the front so that I can hear and see the speaker. Check my notes when I get home to ensure they are useful in the future.

Example 2:

Diabetes update

5 June 2006

Group discussion about case studies

Listening to lecturer talk for a long time

Ask more questions to open up the discussion a little more. Ask for people's contact details so that I can get in touch with them after the event to visit their clinics etc. and see how they work.

Resources for education

Practices receive funding from the nGMS contract to support the continuing development of staff. This support should be specified within the contract of employment. There may also be support for CPD from the PCT, as they have overall responsibility for clinical governance and a duty to support practices with CPD. However, not all PCTs have a separate budget for nurses in general practice, so this should be clarified.

A business case is required when seeking funding for education, and should include the following:

- what the course is
- the cost in terms of fees and time out of the practice
- what would be gained by doing the course
- how it would benefit the practice.

This can then be discussed with the employer.

Sponsorship

Pharmaceutical companies often provide sponsorship for courses pertinent to their products (e.g. in therapy areas such as asthma, chronic obstructive pulmonary disease diploma or degree modules, diabetes). This should be based on an ethical partnership and the practice being happy to accept sponsorship. It is good practice to sign a declaration form detailing what funding is being given and what, if anything, is expected in return.

Scholarships

Sometimes financial awards are granted for educational development. Details of these can be obtained from the Internet or the nursing press. The PCT or health authority may also be aware of opportunities. The following website provides details of educational grants for nurses and HCAs: www.dfes.gov.uk/studentsupport/students/par_part_time_stude.shtml.

Multi-professional training practices

These are a valuable resource, with libraries and regular educational events. They are not always used to develop primary care professionals other than doctors. However, there is no reason why this should be the case, and such practices would provide an ideal opportunity for work-based learning and for training practice nurses.

Individuals

Nurses are increasingly being asked to fund part of their own continuing professional development. Career progression depends on undertaking educational courses to expand knowledge and skills.

Extra information

- Resources for learning – National Electronic Library for Health; www.library.nhs.uk/ Default.aspx
- NHS E-Learning website; www.institute.nhs.uk/learning

Making the most of educational opportunities: nurses

- Some individual practices and/or PCTs run induction programmes for practice nurses. You could ask what happens in your area.
- Some higher education institutions (HEIs) provide undergraduate courses for practice nurses, such as induction modules advancing to the specialist practice degree route, which has general practice nursing as one of its pathways. This culminates in a BSc award and recordable qualification with the NMC. You can find out what your local HEI has to offer by visiting www.hotcourses.com.
- HEIs and other educational establishments offer a wide range of disease-specific modules, leadership modules, and clinical skills and physical assessment modules at a variety of levels to meet individual need. Send for a prospectus to see what they have to offer.
- Nurse prescribing courses can be accessed to help to develop your role further to a high level of autonomy. However, before you are accepted on to a prescribing course you will need to be able to demonstrate skills in assessment linked to NMC standards.[7]
- If you have studied a variety of different modules, you may be able to use the CATS system (see below) to gain a degree or a Master's degree. This is much easier if you study with the same institution.
- Certain PCTs (e.g. Torbay PCT) have developed a structured approach to training and development of practice nurses incorporating formal education for new nurses, ongoing education and support through learning groups for existing nursing staff, and the development of higher-level skills and knowledge to support nurses in achieving special-ist practitioner qualifications. Check whether your PCT has developed such an approach.
- There may be educational opportunities which are run jointly with secondary care (e.g. diabetes or asthma care or refresher study days). Approach clinical nurse specialists to find out whether these are avail-able or whether they will consider running them.
- PCTs or practice nurse forums often run in-house training sessions (e.g. immunisation updates, travel vaccines). Your practice nurse lead for the PCT will be able to tell you how to access these opportunities. If you have difficulty accessing the information, contact the education lead for the PCT.

There is a wide range of opportunities for education and training for practice nurses. It is up to you as an individual to work out your own and your practice's needs and to access the appropriate education and train-ing.

What are CATS points?

The credit accumulation and transfer scheme (CATS) is the HEIs' way of evaluating the academic content of different courses so that points can be collected towards an academic award. Although academic levels are consistent across all HEIs, you will find that they have their own credit ratings for courses, which accumulate as points towards a diploma, degree or Master's degree. Credits from one HEI cannot be automatically transferred to another HEI, but may be included using the APEL method.

What is APEL?

Assessment of prior experiential learning (APEL) is a way of awarding credits for previous learning. Life experiences, professional knowledge and skills are assessed and credited towards a relevant academic course. However, there are some points to remember.

- A professional profile needs to be prepared, which outlines previous learning experiences and the ways in which they have influenced practice.
- Most HEIs charge for APEL assessments, which are complex to administer, so check with the college or university about their system for doing this.
- Assessment of prior learning (APL) allows credit to be awarded for relevant course and examination results.

Example 4.1 Using the APEL and APL procedures in an HEI

Mary is a practice nurse who has worked in practice for about eight years and has been running a COPD (chronic obstructive pulmonary disease) clinic for the last four years. She has enrolled on a degree course at her local university, and when discussing the modules with her tutor shows him a certificate listing the learning outcomes for a 15-credit level 3 COPD module she achieved at another university about four years ago. Mary feels that this together with the considerable experience she has gained in practice should be taken into account when deciding on the most appropriate degree route for her. The tutor explains that the level 3 module at this university is worth 30 credits.

Outcome

The tutor uses the certificate and learning outcomes with the APL system to prove that Mary has undertaken this previous module. In order to complete the other 15 credits at level 3, Mary uses the APEL system to prove that she has undertaken additional learning through managing the patients in the practice. She provides testimonies from her employing GP detailing the level of autonomy she has within the COPD clinic and how effective it has been. She provides evidence (using anonymised clinic sheets) of the number of clinics run, and she completes some reflective writing about the patients she has managed.

All of this evidence will then be taken along to the APEL board for a decision on whether to award 15 credits at level 3 from Mary's prior learning and experience to her current route of studies.

Academic levels of study

You can opt to study at an HEI at various levels. Each university has its own quality assurance systems which are monitored by the Quality Assurance Agency and have their own internal mechanisms for validating programmes. If it is a professional qualification, such as nurse prescribing, these modules will be validated by the NMC.

Level 1

This is equivalent to the first year of study on a normal university course. Anyone who has undertaken an RGN qualification prior to 2000 will have studied at level 1. In order to progress to level 2, you need 120 credits at this level or equivalent (experiential learning).

Level 2

This is equivalent to undergraduate diploma level. You will have achieved this if you have studied Project 2000 and qualified as an RNdipHE. It is equivalent to the second year of a university course.

Many modules at universities are offered at level 2, and you should consider taking these if you have not completed any previous level 2 study (i.e. if you only have basic RGN level). The basic difference is that there is less analysis in the work that you have to undertake.

Level 3

This is equivalent to degree level, and to gain an honours degree you need 120 credits at this level. In order to access level 3 you need either to have 120 credits at level 2 or to prove that you are capable of this level of study (e.g. RGN qualification and ongoing accredited study days).

Most universities offer modular approaches to degrees where each has a certain number of points. Most degree programmes will have compulsory core modules, one of which will be research methods.

Studying at level 3 means that there is more in-depth analysis and critique of research.

Postgraduate diploma

This is intermediate between degree and Master's level study. It is a stop-off point for some people who don't want to do a full Master's dissertation but have studied at level 4.

Level 4

This is equivalent to Master's degree level. In order to access this level you need to have completed a degree or show that you are capable of working at this level through experiential work. Talk to your local university about this.

Master's level study incorporates application of research and the assimilation of new ideas. All Master's degrees will require a dissertation, which is usually research based.

MPhil and PhD

Very few people go on to study at this level. If undertaken, full-time awards may be completed in a minimum of 3 years (or 7 years part-time). This involves research and national networking, and is usually self-directed.

Making the most of educational opportunities: health care assistants

What you need to learn

If you have not done any learning for a long time, you might want to consider enrolling on an Access course at your local college. There are many opportunities for learning and developing your skills within general practice.

Formal learning

Courses, workshops and distance learning packs should all be available. PCTs run courses, but you may have to wait until there are enough HCAs wanting it to justify running it. However, it may sometimes be possible to join courses arranged elsewhere (e.g. a course on recording ECGs for HCAs at the hospital, or on resuscitation with another practice) if you have missed the in-house session at your own practice.

You may be able to join courses for practice. Pharmaceutical companies often fund meetings for nurses who have prescribing responsibilities, and you may be able to join your practice nurse on these where relevant. Many PCTs organise half-days when the whole practice is closed and joins with others for an education session on specified topics.

Case study

Margaret left school at 15 years of age and worked as an office junior until she got married. When the youngest of her three children was five years old, Margaret got a job as a dinner lady. She was still there 15 years later, but then left to look after her mother who was seriously ill. After that, she applied for a job at the surgery as a cleaner and looked after everything, keeping things in good order. Then the practice manager asked her if she would like to become a health care assistant. This came as a bit of a shock, as she had not thought herself capable of working alongside nurses and doctors. With a lot of support from the practice manager, the course tutor and all the staff, she worked through the course arranged by

the PCT. Gradually she began to take over tasks in the surgery from the nurses. Looking back, she thinks she learned something new every day – and still does. Both her parents died from smoking-related diseases and she found herself being angry with people who smoked and were ill as a result of it. Since doing the HCA course, she understands that her beliefs, culture and attitudes made her react like this. Now she can be more constructive in helping people to change. Margaret can hardly believe that she is doing something that she always wished she could do, but never thought she would be capable of doing.
(Buckingham PCT with permission from the County Practice Staff Training and Development Department)

Specific training and education for HCA posts

- **National Vocational Qualifications (NVQs)** are the most well-known qualification for HCAs in general practice. To undertake an NVQ you will need to register with an approved assessment centre. This could be the PCT education department, your local college or a private provider. You will need an assessor, who could be a practice nurse or someone from the assessment centre. An NVQ assesses your competence to undertake a task (i.e. whether you have the necessary knowledge and skills). This means that you will be expected to have undertaken training in the task prior to your assessment.
- **NVQ in Health level 2** is the starting point for HCAs in general practice. This demonstrates that you can undertake a range of clinical activities to an agreed standard.
- **NVQ in Health level 3** enables you to undertake a broader range of clinical activities without direct supervision. This is the required level if you wish to progress to nurse training.

All of the units of competence used within the awards have been developed by the Sector Skills Council, Skills for Health (www.skillsforhealth.org.uk). Each unit focuses on specific activities (e.g. obtaining venous blood samples) and is mapped on to the NHS Knowledge and Skills Framework (NHS KSF).

Foundation degrees are newly emerging awards within universities or colleges, which develop a higher level of skills. Completion of a foundation degree will enable you to work as an Assistant Practitioner. Foundation degrees may give exemption for part of registered nurse training or health-related degrees. Contact your local HEI for further details. Each college or university has its own entry criteria, and you may be asked to undertake a study skills course to prepare for the training. You can obtain more information by visiting www.hotcourses.com.

Other routes for training
Some PCTs have opted to develop their own training schemes. This means that they can organise training to suit local needs, but the disadvantage of these stand-alone courses is that the competences achieved may not be recognised by other PCTs.

- **Open University Diploma** for HCAs in primary care practice level 3. This course provides 60 guided learning hours to underpin the knowledge and skills to develop understanding in clinical settings. Vocationally qualified assessors observe practice and discuss progress with a mentor. The course is backed by the Open University and endorsed by the Qualifications and Curriculum Authority (QCA) (further information can be obtained by contacting vq-awards@open.ac.uk).
- **Primary Care Training Centre**, **Bradford** provides a range of training courses, many of which are tailored to the needs of HCAs in general practice. The majority of these use a distance learning approach. Further information can be obtained by visiting www.primarycaretraining.co.uk.

Education for nurses and HCAs from different perspectives

Employers' perspective

The importance of continuing professional development for general practice nurses and HCAs is paramount for good patient care. The GMS contract emphasises the responsibility of the practice to allow for protected learning time for staff. They need to identify appropriate learning activities and make resources available to develop an optimal learning environment. Patient safety needs to be protected while nurses and HCAs learn and develop.

Strategic perspective

PCTs should consider strategies to help GP employers to release staff for continuing professional development activities and incorporate more learning opportunities, such as providing placement for pre-registration nurses. PCTs should also consider undertaking a training needs analysis in order to identify the needs of nurses and HCAs and to incorporate staff development into wider education and training systems. They should commission appropriate education and ensure that local provision is fit for purpose.

Patient's perspective

It is helpful for patients to have an understanding of the ongoing education and development that is undertaken by nurses in general practice. It is also important to understand that nurses undergo mentorship, and during this time protection of patient confidentiality in clinical learning environments is paramount, together with the need for patient consent (or refusal of consent) to treatment by student nurses.

> **Educationalist's perspective**
>
> Consider liaising with local trusts/GP employers to provide appropriate and attractive education for practice nurses and HCAs. Also consider the advantages of multi-professional education and ways of accrediting and encouraging work-based learning.

Summary

- Education and training are vital components of the development of all nurses and HCAs working in general practice, and should be given due attention within the workplace.
- Learning occurs in different ways, and different people have different ways of learning. The prospect of formal education can induce anxiety, but such learning will ultimately boost confidence.
- Helping individuals to understand their own learning style is important, and can maximise the benefits of education.

References

1   Chambers R, Wakley G, Iqbal Z *et al*. *Prescription for Learning*. Oxford: Radcliffe Medical Press; 2002.

2   United Kingdom Central Council for Nursing, Midwifery and Health Visiting (UKCC). *Position Paper on the Development of the Support Worker Role*. London: UKCC; 1988.

3   Department of Health. *Liberating the Talents*. London: Department of Health; 2002.

4   Nursing and Midwifery Council. *The PREP Handbook*. London: Nursing and Midwifery Council; 2005.

5   Wakley G, Chambers R, Field S. *Continuing Professional Development in Primary Care; making it happen*. Oxford: Radcliffe Medical Press; 2000.

6   Honey and Mumford Learning Styles Questionnaire; www.peterhoney.com/product/brochure

7   Nursing and Midwifery Council. *Standards of Proficiency for Nurse and Midwife Prescribers*. London: Nursing and Midwifery Council; 2006.

5

Professional development and career planning for nurses and health care assistants

This chapter highlights the various career opportunities that are open to nurses and health care assistants working in general practice, and emphasises the importance of structuring a career path with a defined direction. This will ensure that any continuing professional development that is undertaken can help to facilitate future progression.

Introduction

There is a wide range of possible career options for nurses within general practice, and they should consider carefully the skills and background needed for different posts. Career opportunities within general practice nursing will be affected by the individual practice, as the range of roles and responsibilities for nurses vary between practices. This means that some nurses will have to move to another practice in order to advance their career, whereas others may be able to develop into expanded roles within the same practice.

Individuals and employers should think carefully about career planning and professional development. Whether an individual is ambitious or content to stay at a certain level, there will inevitably be times in life when there is a need to move on to something different. For example, a nurse who wants to move into a larger general practice with an excellent reputation will need to demonstrate that they have kept themselves updated – and show how they have used newly acquired skills. Those who want to move into a more advanced position may need to demonstrate that they have undertaken extra study to gain more knowledge, and that they have progressed to an advanced level with proven competence.

Continuing professional development (CPD) is an integral part of quality assurance for all health care workers. The NHS is committed to the concept of lifelong learning, and this is something that should be embraced rather than seen as an encumbrance. This will happen naturally if development activity is directly relevant to the current role.

Career planning

Career planning is vital at all stages of working life. It is about actively seeking and managing opportunities in order to follow a structured pathway in a defined direction. Career planning needs to be done in the context of the likely changes to the way that general practice or the health service in general is organised and changing, through developments such as more patient choice and practice-based commissioning. For instance, the current emphasis on flexible working means that more than one part-time post can be undertaken, maybe working in more than one general practice or having dual clinical and administrative components. Secondment opportunities are becoming more commonplace and varied.

In order to take career analysis a step further, career anchors[1] can be explored. These will help to clarify the meaning and implications of past career decisions and inform future ones using a more in-depth assessment tool. A tool for using career anchors can be found in the online HCA or GPN Toolkit (www.wipp.nhs.uk).

Career planning involves central questions.[2]

- What is the current position?
- What is the desired goal?
- How will this be achieved?
- What will happen if it is not achieved?

In order to have the best chance of succeeding in a career, individuals should:

- appreciate their own values, beliefs and preferences – that is, identify what they want out of work
- recognise any transferable skills, so that strengths can be linked to opportunities
- be flexible about change, to take advantage of career opportunities as they occur
- create an accurate profile that provides a clear picture of strengths and weaknesses both as an individual and as a team member
- identify a career mentor who can provide support in formulating ideas and implementing action plans
- identify opportunities for development, in order to take up progressive learning activities with enough time to learn and practise new skills
- make time and space for reflection on all the above and progress made
- plan for the future – never stop, even if it is to prepare for a fulfilling retirement!

Career plans may focus on developing particular skills and interests within the current post in order to function more effectively. Specialist skills or more variety in the work role may be required. Promotion, with more status, money or responsibility, may be sought. Alternatively, individuals may have reached a stage where other personal pressures in life are just too much on top of a busy job. In this case, it may be worth considering whether more flexible working hours could perhaps improve the work–life balance.

A first step in career planning is to learn more about oneself. Discovering personal strengths, career and job preferences, motivating factors and priorities in life will help to identify direction, and knowing the required balance between work and leisure, and between time and effort, will influence aspirations. Understanding what levels of responsibility, challenge and interaction with other people are required will also contribute to career plans.

Motivating factors

People are motivated by different things. Money, fame and power are all key motivators. Some of the best motivators for fulfilling needs are:

- interesting and/or useful work
- a sense of achievement
- responsibility
- opportunities for career progression or professional development
- gaining new skills or competencies
- a sense of belonging to a practice team or the NHS.

Life experiences, principles and values, relationships with family, friends and colleagues and work identity will all influence career choices. Recognising key drivers for motivation and inspiration may lead to greater self-awareness and more satisfying career choices.

Work values are personal to individuals. That is why it is important to think about what is really wanted and where energy should be focused. A general practice should not direct anyone where they don't wish to go simply in order to suit the practice's needs. Career planning should be firmly in the hands of the individual.

Identifying the positive and negative factors that affect work

In order to gain a wider perspective on current job satisfaction, a force-field analysis could also be undertaken (*see* Tool 5.1).

Tool 5.1 Drawing up a force-field analysis[3]

Draw a horizontal or vertical line in the middle of a sheet of paper. Label one side 'positive' and the other side 'negative.' Draw bars to represent factors that motivate you on the positive side of the line, and factors that are demotivating on the negative side. The thickness and length of the bars should represent the extent of the influence – that is, a short narrow bar will indicate that the positive or negative factor has a minor influence, and a long wide bar will indicate that it has a major effect.

Take an overview of the resulting force-field diagram and consider whether you are content with things as they are, or can think of ways to boost the positive side and minimise the negative factors. You can do this part of the exercise on your own, with a peer or in a small group in your workplace, or with a career mentor or someone from outside your practice. The exercise should help you to realise the extent to which a known influence in your life or in the workplace as a whole is a positive or negative factor. Make a personal action plan to create situations and opportunities to boost the positive factors in your career and minimise the bars on the negative side.

Example of use of a force-field analysis to determine satisfaction with current post as a health care assistant

Positive factors (driving forces)
Career aspirations

Salary

Autonomy

Satisfaction from caring

No uniform

                                          Negative factors (restraining forces)
                                                               Long hours of work

                                                            Demands from patients

                                                                       Job insecurity

                                                               Oppressive hierarchy

Tool 5.2 provides an opportunity for nurses and HCAs to put career planning in context.

Tool 5.2 Undertaking a Life Line Review of your career to date[4]
This is a reflective exercise that requires you to plot (on a timeline) the highs and lows of your career to date and your current post. It is amazing what you can learn about your relative strengths and weaknesses when you look back at how your career path has worked out. Why do you think you can diversify or develop your career now if you have not done so in the past? If your career has been in a rut during some periods in your past, what can you do now to take up the opportunities available and optimise developments for yourself? Adapt the dates on the timeline for yourself. Then write some details of your career to date, reflecting on the positive and negative aspects.

Your timeline

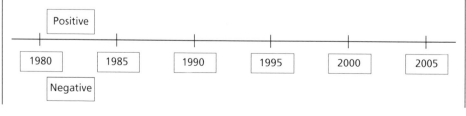

Questions for exploring your timeline experience

- Is there a pattern to the line?
- What do the turning points have in common?
- What types of events were crises for you?

Select a few instances and analyse each of them in depth. What were your circumstances at the time? What were the factors that prevented you from developing your skills or accelerating your career development then? What were the factors that encouraged you or enabled you at the time?
   Ask yourself the following questions.

- What does the line tell you about your attitude to risk?
- Who are the people who have influenced your career to date?
- How have you managed change in your career?
- How would you like the line to look when it is extended to 2010 or 2012?

Having reviewed your career to date, consider what options you now have for career development. Make a plan that takes account of how you have behaved and coped with risk and change in the past.

Learndirect (www.learndirect-advice.co.uk) provides resources for taking stock and evaluating skills from early influences, and making decisions for the future. Their workbook[5] helps to recognise career high and low points, and also to identify the transferable skills and qualities resulting from experience, including the effect of hobbies and leisure activities.

Self-assessment and appraisal

Conducting a self-assessment of strengths, challenges, opportunities and threats relating to career development (*see* Tool 5.3) will provide a clear picture of skills and strengths and will thus help to identify realistic goals.

Tool 5.3 Undertaking a strengths, challenges, opportunities and threats (SCOT) analysis

You can undertake a SCOT analysis of your career working in general practice as an HCA or practice nurse by simply listing the strengths, challenges, opportunities and threats in relation to your role. Work this out either on your own or with the help of a work colleague or mentor.

Strengths might relate to your knowledge or skills, experience, expertise, timekeeping and communication skills.

Challenges may be linked to inter-professional relationships within the team, political factors or personal pressures.

Opportunities might relate to your potential strengths, experience from previous employment that you no longer use, or anticipated changes in the practice.

Threats will include factors and circumstances that prevent you from easily achieving your aims.

List the important factors in your SCOT analysis in order of priority. Once you have done this, draw up goals and a timed action plan for you to achieve your full potential within your career.

Strengths	Challenges
Opportunities	Threats

Appraisal

Individuals need to know what is expected of them within their role in general practice, how they are perceived to have performed, how they are valued as members of the team, and whether there is anything that they could do to improve their performance or to develop their career.

Appraisal is a way of helping both the practice and the individual to grow by helping to consolidate and improve on good performance and identify areas where further development may be necessary. General practice nurses may be required to act as appraisers for HCAs or other junior staff. Similarly, senior HCAs or assistant practitioners may act as appraisers for their junior colleagues.

Appraisal (or individual performance review) should be conducted annually. It is a two-way process, and if conducted in a fair and equitable manner should lead to all staff receiving appropriate development. A personal development plan (PDP) will result from appraisal.

A good appraisal requires adequate preparation by both appraiser and appraisee. Tool 5.4 provides advice and guidance to ensure that appraisals will be of maximum benefit.

Tool 5.4 Effective appraisal

Appraisal is an opportunity to give honest feedback about an individual's performance in order to help them to improve their practice. If you are asked to be an appraiser, take the role seriously and make sure that you have a good understanding of the following:[6]

- the positive and developmental nature of appraisal
- how to prepare for an appraisal
- the structure and process of appraisal
- the stages of an appraisal discussion

- the timetable of the appraisal process
- possible pitfalls
- ground rules
- the qualities that an effective appraiser should possess
- the scope of appraisal and what distinguishes the role of an appraiser from other work-related roles
- how to overcome problems and constraints that might crop up during an appraisal discussion.

An effective appraiser will:

- use description rather than judgement
- keep it friendly, both verbally and non-verbally
- identify and reinforce strengths
- precisely define and mutually agree on problems
- collect objective evidence
- collaborate on constructive solutions
- identify and use 'carrots and sticks' to make it happen
- not capitulate on the standards.

Here are some guidelines for the appraisal process.[7]

- The appraisee and appraiser need to meet regularly. In the best schemes, progress is reviewed frequently. Annual reviews are often recommended but are generally insufficient.
- Nothing should come as a shock at a formal appraisal interview. Ongoing feedback should be a regular feature in people's everyday work in the NHS.
- Appraisal is not a substitute for day-to-day supervision, support and feedback on performance.
- Appraisers have an ongoing responsibility to ensure that the people they appraise can achieve the agreed objectives and where necessary give or direct them to help.
- The appraisee plays the major part in setting objectives, but these must be set within the overall framework of what staff in their post and grade are expected to achieve or demonstrate.
- Self-assessment is an important part of appraisal, but the appraiser must curb the tendency of individuals who are being appraised to be unreasonably self-critical.
- Appraisal interviews should be conducted on a one-to-one basis.
- Confidentiality should be respected. The only exception to this is where poor performance is threatening patient safety. The appraiser has a professional responsibility to protect patients, and this exception should be made explicit at the start of the appraisal process.

Preparing for the appraisal session as an appraiser[6-8]

As an appraiser, it is important that you are at least as well prepared for each meeting as the individuals whom you are appraising. It is your responsibility to set an agenda and guide the meeting. Figure 5.1 provides you with a structure for the meeting. A relaxed atmosphere is crucial, but it is equally important not to spend too much time chatting before you move on to the purpose of the appraisal meeting.

Remember that issues should be explored from the perspectives both of the appraisee and of the practice, the PCT or the NHS as a whole. Keep clarifying what is being said so that you both share the same perspectives, and to obtain a full picture. At the end of the meeting it is important that the actions are agreed by both of you.

At the appraisal

- Create an informal and relaxed atmosphere and put the appraisee at ease.
- Explain the purpose and timing of the appraisal meeting and what outcomes you expect.
- Agree the 'ground rules', including any limits set on confidentiality (such as the belief that patient safety may be at risk).
- Go through your agenda and invite the appraisee to add their own points.
- Explain that you will be taking notes, and what will happen to your records.
- Encourage the appraisee to review their performance as you talk through the achievements of their last year's PDP.
- Let the appraisee do most of the talking.
- Follow your pre-prepared structure, but be flexible and vary the timing according to the other person's needs.
- Points to consider during the appraisal include national and local priorities, review of any significant event analysis, review of audits and protocol developments, review of prescribing data and referral data, working relationships with colleagues, feedback from or involvement with patients, last year's PDP and goals set there.
- Discuss the appraisee's performance, focusing on facts and avoiding subjective judgements. You could structure discussion around the three domains of knowledge, skills and attitudes, or the core competencies of the individual's specialty, discipline or post.
- Give feedback by emphasising the positive aspects and encouraging the appraisee to reflect on and value their achievements.
- Discuss any areas where their performance could have been improved and why. Issues may be personal or operational or relate to the limited availability of resources or training opportunities.
- Discuss possible career paths or first steps and how the appraisee views them.
- Jointly agree the objectives for a future personal development plan based on the appraisal discussion.
- Jointly agree what training and development needs have been identified, and encourage the appraisee to make a realistic plan.
- Summarise what has been agreed – the appraisee going first and you as appraiser afterwards reaffirming, revising or adding to what they have

said. Reinforce their strengths and opportunities, and the ways you have jointly identified for them to resolve problems and address their needs.
- Agree their plan for the future.
- Agree the next steps (the timescale for writing up documentation, an interim review date, the next appraisal date, etc.). Some appraisers organise the appraisal session so that they have a short break in which to reflect at the end of the appraisal, then complete the paper records and share this report with the appraisee.

After the appraisal

- Complete the paperwork, and share a copy with the individual you have appraised.
- Feed back appraisal information in an anonymous way to the primary care organisation in order to inform its planning process. It may be that the clinical governance lead in your trust or organisation has a central role in this process, collating appraisal information from the entire workforce to inform the organisation's various strategies.
- Organise an interim review as appropriate (a phone call to check on progress or resolution of issues, a face-to-face meeting for more substantial concerns, etc.).

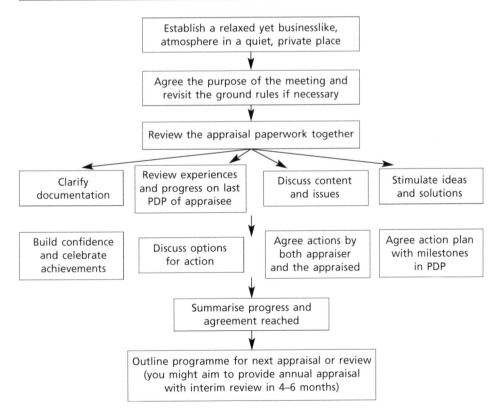

Figure 5.1 The process of the appraisal meeting, from the appraiser's perspective

Personal development plans

Developing a personal development plan helps to consolidate thoughts, and should be completed following appraisal. If the employer reads it, everyone will be aware of its long- and short-term aspirations.

Case study

Linda records in her personal development plan (PDP) that she is often asked for information leaflets on subjects such as hypertension, cholesterol and immunisation as part of her role as an HCA. She has to tell patients to ask the nurse or doctor for leaflets. She has talked about this in her HCA forum that meets every three months, and finds that another HCA prints out the patient information leaflets (PILS) from the link to PRODIGY on the computer. At the review of her PDP, Linda discusses how she could learn to print out PILS to benefit patients and reduce the work of the nurse and doctor. The practice manager arranges an in-house session to help her to find her way around Prodigy and learn how to print out information leaflets. Linda makes a record of the instructions for this activity and keeps this in her folder with her PDP. Over the next three months she keeps a record of which leaflets she prints out to demonstrate that she is competent at this new skill and that it is relevant to her post.

Tool 5.5 Drafting your personal development plan

This simple example will help you to formulate your ideas for a personal development plan.

Making a draft personal development plan

Your needs:
How you can meet those needs:
How you will know when you have met those needs:

What are the challenges in your job now that you need to meet?

Where do you want to be in two years' time?

Where do you want to be in five or ten years' time?

How does that fit in with what the practice wants?

What adjustments will you need to make in order to achieve what you want?

What adjustments will other people need to make, for you to achieve what you want?

What else should you consider?

Personal development plan template

The PDP can be completed to individual specification so long as it contains the minimum content and scope specified here.

Time span to which it relates:

Date last updated:

Topics prioritised in PDP for the previous year:

Justify why current topics in PDP are a priority:

Is this linked to any personal or professional priorities?

Is this linked to any practice or team priorities?

Is this linked to any national drivers to improve health care?

What else will be included in your PDP?

What baseline information will you collect and how? How will you identify your learning needs?

What are the learning needs for the practice or team and how do they match your needs?

Is there any patient or public input to your PDP?

What are the aims of your PDP arising from the preliminary data-gathering exercise?

Action plan (give tasks, timetable, endpoints, etc.)

How does your PDP tie in with your other strategic plans (e.g. the practice's business or development plan)?

What additional resources will you require to execute your plan and where will you find them? (Will you have to pay any course fees? Will you be able to organise any protected time for learning during working hours?)

How will you evaluate your PDP?

How will you know when you have achieved your objectives? (How will you measure success?)

How will you disseminate the learning from your plan to the rest of the practice/PCT team and patients? How will you sustain your new-found knowledge or skills?

How will you handle new learning requirements as they arise?

Record sheet to describe progress in work-based learning

Record your discussions, your action plan, your resource requirements and the outcomes that you expect. Think how you will collect evidence that demonstrates you have achieved what you have planned. Use the form below to record these aspects of your problem-based learning sessions.

Your priority topic:

Where you are now:

What you do next includes:

What extra resources might this require?

The outcomes might include:

How would you demonstrate that you have achieved your outcomes?

Mentorship

As most nurses and HCAs are employed in a practice, they have to work hard at establishing networks that will provide support and ideas. They may suffer from professional isolation, which could lead to lack of motivation or failure to identify career opportunities. Therefore it is advisable to find a mentor. A mentor's role is to provide advice and guidance, and to act as a sounding board to rehearse ideas or responses to challenges. Mentorship will ensure that there is time to stop and focus on current direction, development needs and whether objectives have been identified. A mentor needs to have insight into the variety and opportunities that exist within general practice nursing, and should be someone to whom it is easy to relate. It is probably not a good idea to select the line manager or GP employer, because of potential conflict of interests. A mentoring relationship is primarily a one-way relationship in which the mentor has the time and capacity to listen and help to make career-related decisions. Some mentors are only concerned with helping the mentee to identify and meet their educational or training needs through a development plan, whereas others give practical or emotional support as well.

The emphasis is on the mentor helping the mentee to develop their own thinking and find their own way, not on teaching the mentee new skills or acting as a patron to ease the mentee's career path by giving them special favours.

A mentor helps the mentee to realise their potential by acting as a trusted senior counsellor and experienced guide on personal, professional and educational matters. A mentor should be able to agree learning objectives with the mentee and subsequently guide them to address their educational needs, identify their strengths and weaknesses, explore options with them, act as a challenger, encourage reflection and provide motivation. The relationship between mentor and mentee should be one of mutual trust and respect – a supportive yet challenging relationship which remains non-judgemental.

Tool 5.6 Effective mentorship

At the start of a mentoring relationship, ground rules should be agreed for meetings, including confidentiality, commitment, duration and frequency of sessions, location, purpose, personal boundaries and how or whether you will record your meeting. Clarify the objectives and outcomes that you both want to cover. A common framework[9] used for mentoring follows three stages.

1 **Exploration.** The mentor listens, and prompts the mentee with questions.
2 **New understanding.** The mentor listens and challenges the mentee, recognises the strengths and weaknesses of the ideas, shares experiences, establishes priorities, identifies development needs, and gives information and supportive feedback.
3 **Action planning.** The mentor encourages new ways of thinking, and helps the mentee to reach a solution, agree goals and decide on action plans.

A mentor and mentee may be from different backgrounds, and the differences may provoke a cross-fertilisation of ideas and shared understanding and perspectives. The mentoring session may be an opportunity to reinforce or analyse what learning took place after performing a new task or activity, such as a secondment.

Continuing professional development

Continuing professional development (CPD) can be defined as:

> a process of lifelong learning for all individuals and teams which meets the needs of patients and delivers the health outcomes and health care priorities of the NHS and which enables professionals to expand and fulfil their potential.[10]

A new framework for CPD was set out in *A First Class Service*[11] and in the Chief Medical Officer's review of CPD in general practice.[10] The challenge set by the framework is not to develop new ways of learning in primary care, but rather to put in place a management process that will support CPD that is undertaken and make it evidence based and relevant.

Learning and development is an ongoing process, and the more that skills and knowledge can be developed, the more roles can be widened.

Many areas provide support groups for nurses in general practice where they can meet and exchange ideas, discuss problems and provide support for each other. Many groups also invite speakers to talk about certain aspects of health care relevant to the clinical work in general practice. Tool 5.7 gives guidance on how to set up a support forum.

Tool 5.7 Setting up a forum for nurses and HCAs in general practice

Here are a few suggestions for setting up a network forum for nurses and HCAs working in general practice.

- Make a list of key people to help form a group. These may include the PCT professional lead for practice nurses/HCAs, nurses from general practice who are well known in the local area, and a lecturer in general practice nursing/NVQ trainer.
- Contact pharmaceutical companies for sponsorship for hiring a venue or supplying refreshments. To avoid the possibility of bias, take sponsorship from different companies throughout the year.
- Find out whether a local practice will allow the group to meet on its premises in the evening.
- Draw up a list of topics for 12 months, and ask practice nurses and HCAs to comment on them.
- Ask GPs and other health care professionals for advice on expert speakers in different areas.
- Set up, or ask the PCT to set up, a password-protected discussion board for members on the PCT website, to encourage the sharing of good practice.
- Plan a monthly meeting that could take place at the same time as other community nurse meetings and include some training updates. This should take place within normal working hours and be seen as part of CPD.
- Set up an email group to share information.

To make the forum meetings successful, remember the following main points.

- Someone with an interest in developing nursing in general practice will need to take charge of coordinating the meetings. This could be the PCT professional lead or any nurse who has good contacts throughout the local area.
- Arrange for discussion topics to be advertised in advance. These need to be interesting, interactive and current.
- Keep a record of what has been discussed and any training given, and add this information to your personal/professional development portfolio as evidence of professional updating.

The Royal College of Nursing provides a specialist forum for nurses in general practice (www.rcn.org.uk/members/yourspeciality/newsletter-plus/forum/index.php?fd=practicenurses).

Effective CPD involves identifying educational needs, learning in a variety of different ways, and implementing and reinforcing that learning. This should therefore be supported with an allowance for study time, mentorship and support within practices. Tool 5.8 considers the features that practices should include within a policy for study leave.

Tool 5.8 What to look for in a study leave policy

A study leave policy should ensure that everyone has equal opportunities and access to study leave, and that such leave is given in an appropriate and equal manner. The practice should also provide some framework and record of all study leave. This will highlight areas of excellence within the practice and areas of deficit which need to be developed.

There will be local variation depending on the size and location of the practice, but a good study leave policy should:

• allow time for CPD. This should be in addition to time allowed for mandatory updating (e.g. cardiopulmonary resuscitation training) determined by the PCT
• be calculated on a pro-rata basis with an equal entitlement for all members of staff (e.g. five days). An exception would be a specific course or qualification that requires more days to complete (e.g. nurse prescribing, which includes a statutory 26 days' tuition)
• link study leave to the practice objectives; this may mean only allowing attendance on courses and study days that are directly relevant for the practice. The needs and development of the individual should also be linked via the creation of a personal development plan (*see* page 74)
• include guidance on where to obtain funding for the study-leave event (e.g. state whether there is a practice education budget, or whether the PCT funds training and development).

Clinical supervision

Clinical supervision is the sharing of ideas and events in practice, and it contributes to lifelong learning. Nurses analyse and learn from real-life events in practice, and consider whether these have been dealt with appropriately or whether they could have been managed more effectively in another way. Clinical supervision supports practice and should therefore be encouraged by employers.

The benefits of clinical supervision are that it:

• encourages learning through shared reflection
• provides support and reduces stress
• provides alternative ideas and new ways of looking at issues
• reduces professional isolation
• enhances job satisfaction and thus improves retention.

Case study: The value of clinical supervision

Lynda has worked as a practice nurse for two years. She enjoys her job but finds it stressful at times, and has frequently considered leaving to join the district nursing service, where she feels that support and teamwork are more pronounced.

The professional lead for practice nursing persuades Lynda to attend a local clinical supervision support group. This is a group of five practice nurses who have been meeting together for 1½ hours once a month for the last year. The group is facilitated by the professional lead, and is held in a different practice each month. The group members have established ground rules to suit themselves about the nature of their sessions, and understand that the principles of confidentiality apply to all of their discussions. Lynda was invited in as a new member, and agreed to attend each month unless there was a very genuine reason why she could not do so. She also agreed not to divulge details of any incidents discussed in the group to other people.

Lynda wasn't sure what to expect at her first meeting, so she spent the first hour listening to others talk about events or situations which had occurred that had caused them some upset or anxiety. She found that she was able to identify with many of the situations discussed, and that she was able to offer some good advice on how she had tackled similar situations in the past. She then talked about one of the GPs she worked with whom she felt was constantly challenging her and belittling her. As she talked about this she realised what a relief it was to be able to voice some of her concerns, but she also learned that others interpreted some of the GP's actions quite differently – she began to realise that this challenging approach could be regarded as the GP being interested in her development, and that it was a way of building confidence and trust. The group suggested a variety of ways to tackle this behaviour and she agreed to put these into practice and report back.

The following month Lynda was pleased to share with the group that the situation had improved dramatically and that she felt much better about herself for having tackled the situation. She was already feeling more confident, and the sessions enabled her to feel genuinely supported by her peers in a way that she had never experienced within general practice, where there were only two nurses, who found it difficult to admit their mistakes to each other.

Overcoming barriers to clinical supervision in general practice

Clinical supervision requires protected time and commitment both from participating nurses and from employers. Meeting with other nurses or HCAs from general practice can provide a valuable insight into different ways of working, but may also appear threatening to employers if they don't understand the concept of clinical supervision. If there is currently no time allowed for clinical supervision in a practice, it is important to make sure that the benefits are fully understood by employers, and using real-life examples may demonstrate how practice has been changed. It is often easier to hold clinical supervision sessions away from the practice in order to avoid constant interruptions. Tool 5.9 provides tips to help to make the introduction of clinical supervision successful.

Tool 5.9 Clinical supervision: how to make it work

Identify a suitable venue and dates and book this in advance.

The venue needs to be private, but could be within a GP surgery or health centre. Any phones would need to be re-routed for the duration of the meeting.

Determine the length and frequency of meetings.
The length of meetings needs to be at least two hours if there is a group format, to allow for meaningful discussion. Monthly or 6-weekly meetings are most likely to be supported by employers. More frequent meetings are less likely to be supported.

Clarify the role of supervisors.
This is likely to include coordination of sessions, establishing and maintaining ground rules, establishing a 'safe' environment, facilitation of the process, summary and action planning, and documentation.

Identify potential supervisors and determine training needs.
Supervisors need to be skilled and experienced practitioners. They must be good listeners who are able to provide constructive feedback and be open and tolerant of others. They need to have had training in reflective practice, law and accountability, self-awareness, group dynamics and supervision practice.

Establish a method for supervising the supervisors.
Supervisors may have to provide considerable emotional support and take on board issues that cause concern or anxiety. It is therefore essential for them to be able to receive support and debriefing in a formal way.

Ensure that the PCT is involved in the planning and maintenance of this initiative.
PCTs will have experience of managing clinical supervision sessions for their community nursing staff, and are therefore well placed to advise and support general practice nurses.

Ensure that GPs are aware of the benefits of and need for clinical supervision.
In order for GPs to support general practice nurses' time out of practice, they need to appreciate the potential that clinical supervision has for improving practice. The PCT may have a link role in this.

Use a framework within supervision sessions.
This will provide a structure to ensure that the process is meaningful and to make participants feel more secure.

For more detailed information, see www.wipp.nhs.uk.

Career development from the general practice nursing perspective

The plethora of job titles and variety of roles pose challenges to practices in terms of defining jobs and levels of practice. Outlining the roles on the basis of the activities that practice nurses do, rather than relying on job titles to differentiate between roles, is one way forward. This is the principle underlying the Knowledge and Skills Framework[12] that seeks to:

- clarify what knowledge and skills are needed in a post
- accurately apply knowledge and skills to job demands
- ensure access to appropriate learning and development
- identify the knowledge and skills needed for career progression
- link appropriate pay to appropriate use of knowledge and skills.

Even if the practice you work for has not yet adopted *Agenda for Change*,[13] it is still worth looking at the Knowledge and Skills Framework. This consists of six core dimensions, which you will do in your job at a defined level. There are 24 other specific dimensions, some of which you will do at varying levels depending on the nature of your role and responsibilities as a practice nurse. The Knowledge and Skills Framework job profiles will act as a prompt for action by you and your manager at your annual appraisal, to ensure that your knowledge and skills with regard to your current job are up to date. You will review your opportunity for personal and professional development. This may be to complement the work you currently undertake or to prepare you for another role to help you progress in your career. It will also enable you to see what knowledge and skills are required for future career steps, and to identify the development you will need to support your progress on your career path.

The current array of titles used within general practice nursing can be confusing for both you and your employer. Some PCTs and health authorities have created definitions of these terms to provide local clarity. In addition, the RCN has set definitions for the titles of advanced nurse practitioner and specialist nurse (see www.rcn.org.uk). The NMC has also provided a defined level of preparation for an advanced nurse practitioner (see www.nmc-uk.org).

Using the nationally approved framework 'General Practice Nursing Career Pathway' will provide clarity and create consistency.

Advanced nursing practice

The title of advanced nurse practitioner will soon be formally recognised by the NMC for nurses who have undertaken significant advanced-level study to reach a defined level, usually Master's degree level. Often these nurses will also be able to prescribe. Nurses using this title will be trained to undertake physical examination and manage many conditions autonomously. The NMC is planning to record this title as an additional component on the register. Once this happens there will be a transient period of three years during which time existing nurse practitioners can improve their skills to the requisite level to register with the NMC as advanced nurse practitioners.

Nurses who use the title 'nurse practitioner' will be unable to do so after the transition period has ended. Current nurse practitioners will need to prove to their professional regulatory body that they have the requisite skills to be registered as advanced nurse practitioners, or undertake further study to progress to this stage.

Apprenticeship schemes

Some PCTs are developing apprenticeship schemes which provide the basic education and training to enable an individual nurse to work within general practice. Successful completion of the course puts the individual in a good position to move up the career ladder as a general practice nurse. Some practices and PCTs now stipulate this as a mandatory requirement.

Practice nurse facilitators

A practice nurse facilitator/adviser can be an invaluable asset to the education and training of nurses working in general practice who are employed within the PCT. This role needs to be clearly defined, and must have the support and backing of the PCT so that the individual has the authority to put in place training sessions and help staff to be released from their workplace to attend training and educational events, whether in-house or at local universities.

The role is invaluable for keeping records up to date about the training and educational needs of the nurses working in general practice within the PCT, and also for highlighting where excellent care is being provided so that this can be utilised for the training and supervision of other practice nurses who are in training in certain areas.

Role expansion

As many practice nurses are expanding their roles to take on more work that has traditionally been managed by GPs (e.g. management of long-term conditions within nurse-led clinics), it is vital that nurses do not feel coerced into taking on extra responsibilities without appropriate education. Registered nurses must not take on a new role or task if they or their employer do not consider that they are competent to do so without breaching the *Code of Professional Conduct*[14] and being open to a charge of professional misconduct. There are two legal standards that apply to the expansion of nurses' roles. The first is a 'constitutional stand' (the rule of law), which requires the nurse to act within the law. The second is a minimum quality standard (the rule of negligence), which requires a nurse who takes on a role or task previously performed by a doctor, for example, to perform that task or role to the same standard as a doctor. It is essential that nurses who take on any new role are aware of the legal boundaries relating to the role, and that they have sufficient training and preparation to ensure that they can perform the role to the required standard.

Future roles for practice nurses

Although role development can be seen in terms of advancing to a lead general practice nurse or advanced nurse practitioner, a further option of nurse partner is available. New initiatives[15,16] point to nurses becoming partners in a practice and providing additional services such as out-of-hours care. The benefits and challenges of becoming a nurse partner can be summarised as follows.

Benefits:

- autonomy and independence
- being involved in decision making/strategic planning at a higher level
- greater patient advocacy
- significantly higher pay achieved through profit sharing
- wider opportunities to develop their career
- greater job satisfaction
- better teamwork.

Challenges:

- knowing about employment law
- understanding and handling finances
- sorting out pension and insurance issues
- long irregular hours
- changing relationships with nursing and medical colleagues
- financial investment in the practice.

More information on becoming a nurse partner can be found at www.london.nhs.uk/Iscn/publications/Nurse-Partner-Factsheet.pdf

Another area of development is the advent of the Practitioner with a Special Interest[17] (PwSI). This role supplements a generalist role by delivering a high-quality, improved-access service to meet the needs of a PCT or a group of PCTs. PwSIs may deliver a clinical service beyond the normal scope of general practice, undertake advanced procedures or develop services. There are numerous PwSIs employed by PCTs in different areas of clinical care.

The following is a quote from a nurse with a special interest in diabetes:

'The services we offer are very patient-centred. Our clinics are local, easy to access, and give patients the confidence of knowing they can see someone they know who has the time to spend with them. We don't diagnose. Our role is to troubleshoot, advise, support and educate.'

Case study: Career progression within general practice nursing

After working as a health visitor for several years I decided that I missed the 'hands-on' nursing within nursing. I was looking for part-time work, and when a post in practice nursing was advertised at a local practice, I decided to apply for it. I think I got the job because I was skilled at making good relationships with families and I could demonstrate that I could work without direct supervision and was good at organising my workload. When I started the job I was astounded at the variety of work and the pace that I needed to work at. If it hadn't been for the support of other, experienced practice nurses in the team, I would have left within the first few weeks because I felt so overwhelmed! I attended an introductory course for new practice nurses run by the local university, and this really helped to lift my confidence and competence.

The GPs I worked with then asked if I would set up a weight control clinic, as they recognised the need for this within the practice. This was successful, and I attended a course on obesity management and nutrition, which developed my knowledge further. Many of the patients attending the clinic had diabetes, so my interest in this area also increased, but I recognised that my knowledge was scanty. I approached one of the GPs I worked with who had a special interest in diabetes, and asked if he would help me to learn more. We had tutorials once a fortnight when I would discuss patients and we would go through their management. I booked myself on a Diabetes module at the local university, and during this time set up a diabetes clinic which I ran, with the doctor being available for help and advice. It wasn't long before my knowledge matched up to his and I was able to make the clinic nurse-led. I have since undertaken audits looking at the care of patients with diabetes, and am pleased to say that the care and control have improved significantly since I have been actively following up patients. I undertook the nurse prescribing course so that I can now prescribe for my patients. The PCT ask me to speak at various education events, and I am a designated support nurse for other practice nurses who want to set up diabetes clinics. This means that I attend their surgeries and work with them to determine appropriate management for patients. I also teach on the Diabetes module at the university, where I talk about the practical issues involved in setting up diabetes clinics in general practice. I am now employed as a senior-grade practice nurse with a special interest in diabetes. I love my role and never stop learning!

Tool 5.10 can be used as a discussion tool to define the roles of nurses in general practice. The roles outlined within this tool are examples, and are likely to be subject to local variation.

Tool 5.10 Varying roles within general practice nursing

This tool provides examples of different roles and job titles. Devise a local interpretation of roles after discussing these with PCTs and practices.

Role:

Outline of typical activities:

Qualifications that may be required:

Experience that is likely to be required:

Local PCT or practice interpretation and title for this role and any additional activities included:

Basic-grade HCA
Venepuncture, screening of height, weight and blood pressure, urine testing, administrative duties.

No formal qualification required, but basic skills in literacy and numeracy necessary; may hold NVQ level 2 or be working towards NVQ level 3. Life experience, dealing with the public, experience of caring.

Senior-grade HCA
As above, plus ECG recording, health promotion activities and advice giving, simple wound care, assisting in minor surgery, stock control.
NVQ level 3, or working towards this.
Experience working as a basic-grade HCA.

Assistant/associate practitioner
As above, plus skills that require some assessment (e.g. ear syringing, immunisation, advice giving).
Foundation degree, or working towards this.
Experience working as a senior-grade HCA.

General practice nurse
Wide range of duties common within general practice nursing (e.g. health promotion and advice, dressings, ear syringing, vaccinations).
RGN.*
Some post-registration general nursing experience usually required.

Senior general practice nurse
As above, plus cervical cytology screening, running nurse-led clinics (with some GP involvement), undertaking clinical audit.
RGN.* Accredited course in general practice nursing or accredited course in disease-specific management[†] (e.g. asthma, diabetes).
Experience of practice nursing required.

Lead general practice nurse
As above, plus team leadership, nurse-led care (without routine GP intervention), first-contact care (with some GP involvement).
RGN.* Accredited degree-level course in practice nursing[†] (e.g. BSc Hons Specialist Practice – GPN).
Minimum of two years of practice nurse experience usually required.

Advanced nurse practitioner
As above, plus leading on creation of practice policies, clinical guidelines, etc.; first-contact care (without routine GP intervention); clinical teaching for junior staff/medical students.
RGN.* Honours degree or higher degree relating to clinical nursing.[†] Extended/supplementary prescribing qualification, leadership qualification.[†]
Minimum of three years of practice nurse experience. Competence in clinical examination and assessment.

Nurse partner
Clinical activity highly variable, but involves investment in a practice,

income generation, proportionate share in profits together with share in decision making relating to the practice.

RGN.* Knowledge of financial systems in general practice.†

Minimum of two years of practice nurse experience usually required.

Practice nurse facilitator/developer

Works across practices to support the development of practice nurses. Involved in mentorship and educational activities for practice nurses.

RGN.* First degree in practice nursing† (e.g. BSc Hons Specialist Practice – GPN).

Minimum of two years of practice nurse experience usually required.

Practice nurse professional lead

Provides advice and guidance to the PCT or Strategic Health Authority on professional issues, and may be responsible for performance management/clinical governance relating to practice nurses.

RGN.* First degree in nursing or general practice nursing† (e.g. BSc Hons Specialist Practice – Practice Nursing). Higher degree, leadership qualification.†

Minimum of three years of practice nurse experience.

Specialist practice nurse

Runs nurse-led clinics in a specific disease area (e.g. coronary heart disease), provides advice and guidance to the practice on creation of guidelines and policies relating to this area, designs and undertakes clinical audit; provides education for other practice nurses and community nurses.

RGN.* First degree in nursing or general practice nursing.† Accredited course in disease-specific management* (e.g. asthma, diabetes), basic-level teaching/mentorship qualification.†

Minimum of three years of practice nurse experience.

Lecturer in general practice nursing

Designs and delivers education programmes for practice nurses; inputs education relating to practice nurse role into pre-registration nursing programmes.

RGN.* First degree in nursing or general practice nursing† (e.g. BSc Hons Specialist Practice – practice nursing). Higher degree.† Teaching qualification.†

Minimum of three years of practice nurse experience.

Head of general practice nurse education

Identifies development needs for practice nurses and directs programme development; manages practice nurse lecturers, liaison with PCTs, workforce development directorates and deaneries.

Higher degree.† Teaching qualification.†

Experience in practice nursing required.

* Essential † Highly desirable.

Career development from the health care assistant's perspective

The potential of HCAs working in general practice is only just being realised.[18] That is, the numbers employed and the hours per week for which they are employed are limited, as are the roles and responsibilities that HCAs are asked to take on. A few practices and PCTs support HCAs in their career progression to more senior HCA roles or to gain nursing and allied health professional registration qualifications, but at the moment they are the exception rather than the rule. Career progression has been made easier by NVQs, the qualifications underpinning HCA training, as they are based on National Occupational Standards, and therefore provide a benchmark of competence. Although NVQs provide a national standard, many registered nurses may not be conversant with the requirements for these awards. This can pose a problem for HCAs in general practice, but it can be overcome by speaking to the PCT professional lead/practice nurse facilitator, who is likely to have a broader understanding of the competences and supervision required.

Assistant practitioners

This new role (discussed in Chapter 1) provides an option for HCAs who wish to develop further but who do not want to access registered nurse training. An integral part of the development of this role is work-based training. This is completed by a foundation degree, at level 4 of the National Qualification Framework.[19] This is a higher education qualification worth 240 credits, and it usually takes two to three years to complete. A foundation degree is validated by a university and delivered in partnership with further education colleges. It gives learners a combination of technical, vocational, academic and transferable skills, and is an important step on the Career Framework[20] between NVQ level 3 and full professional training.

Moving on to registered nurse training

Achievement of NVQ level 3 generally provides access to general nurse training if this is required, and foundation degrees may provide exemption from the common foundation programme in general nurse training in some areas. You will need to check with your local university whether this is the case in your area.

Some Health Authorities may provide financial sponsorship for HCAs who have NVQ level 3, so it is worth enquiring whether this is the case in your area. You could also ask the practice you work for if they would be prepared to support you while you undertake nurse training. If you do wish to access registered nurse training, financial support for eligible students is available in the form of an NHS bursary. The grant is awarded to you to cover everyday living costs, such as accommodation, and depends on the level of undergraduate course (diploma or degree) that you opt for (see www.nhscareers.nhs.uk/nhs-knowledge_base/data/225.html).

Progressing along your career path

Have a look at the Skills for Health career framework,[20] which has the nine key elements listed in Table 5.2. This will help you to envisage how your HCA post fits in with the hierarchy of the map of all NHS careers.

Key elements of the Career Framework[20]

- **Level 9. More senior staff** – with ultimate responsibility for clinical caseload decision making and full on-call accountability.
- **Level 8. Consultant practitioners** – staff working at a very high level of clinical expertise and/or with responsibility for planning of services.
- **Level 7. Advanced practitioners** – experienced clinical professionals with a very high standard of skills and knowledge.
- **Level 6. Senior practitioners/specialist practitioners** – staff with a higher degree of autonomy and responsibility than 'practitioners.'
- **Level 5. Practitioners** – most frequently registered practitioners in their first and second post-registration/professional qualification jobs.
- **Level 4. Assistant practitioners/associate practitioners** – deliver protocol-based clinical care under the direction and supervision of a state-registered practitioner. Probably studying for or attained a foundation degree, BTEC higher or HND.
- **Level 3. Senior health care assistants/technicians** – have a higher level of responsibility than a support worker. Probably studying for or attained NVQ level 3 or Assessment of Prior Experiential Learning (APEL).
- **Level 2. Support workers** – frequently have the job title of 'health care assistant' or 'health care technician.' Probably studying for or attained NVQ level 2.
- **Level 1. Initial entry level jobs** – such as domestic assistants or cadets requiring very little formal education or previous knowledge, skills or experience in delivering or supporting the delivery of health care.

You can look on the Skills for Health website (www.skillsforhealth.org.uk/careerframework/tools.php) to review the career pathways that are available to all NHS staff. You could use this career tool to find out what career options are available to you relating to your personal and practice commitments. For instance, a senior health care assistant has several career options at level 4 if they continue to develop their competence (an assistant practitioner in radiography or nursing, or a community care assistant). Tameside and Glossop PCT has introduced trainee assistant practitioners who provide invaluable assistance to other health care professionals while receiving training on the job.

Others, such as Pat in the case study below, progress to level 5 after they have gained a professional qualification at university as a nurse or allied health professional. Pat's experience demonstrates the route that a health care assistant could take to progress in their career – from receptionist to health care assistant to registered nurse. Her general practice employers supported her throughout in undertaking basic training and then an NVQ in care. Even when she became a full-time student nurse, the practice kept in touch with her and provided support. They hope that there will be a vacancy for her as a practice nurse in the future, if she chooses nursing in a primary care setting for the next stage of her career.

If you are unsure about the career route that you want to pursue, have a look at the website www.nhscareers.nhs.uk. It gives easy access to career guidance for all types of NHS careers. You can then consult the experts in careers at your PCT about the various options that are available and any funding that is available. You can also search for appropriate courses at your local universities and colleges and check their individual entry requirements.

Case study: Progression from receptionist to health care assistant to registered nurse at the Ridge Medical Practice, Bradford

'Pat' had been a receptionist in the practice for a number of years when she expressed an interest in becoming a health care assistant. She applied for a vacant post on the nursing team. She was duly appointed and commenced her induction period. Following this, Pat undertook phlebotomy training at the local hospital and began to settle into her new role. She then commenced a university-accredited primary care HCA course (for example, see www.primarycaretraining.com), which she completed six months later. A further period of consolidation followed in which Pat undertook ECG and spirometry training, and her role expanded to include other duties such as assisting in minor surgery, interviewing new patients and working alongside the practice nurses in the cardiovascular and diabetes chronic disease management clinics.

Twelve months later Pat had successfully completed her NVQ level 3 in Care, and it was tremendously rewarding to see how she was developing in her role. The nurse team leader felt that she had additional potential, and encouraged her to consider nurse training. She applied for a place at the local university school of nursing, and is now a full-time first-year student nurse. The practice will continue to support Pat during her study. They have set up an agreement which will enable her to keep in contact and access any practice information which may help in her studies, including audit facilities and the practice library.

Case study: The Hanham Surgery

The Hanham Surgery reports that:

Both our existing HCAs were initially employed as receptionists. They have gradually developed their role from part-time phlebotomists/receptionists to their current roles as full-time, integrated members of the nursing team. They have a wide range of competences and have been key to enabling the practice to meet access targets by shifting work to the most appropriate practitioner and freeing up nurse time to manage the chronic disease element of patient care. In their own right they have worked holistically with the rest of the team to ensure that all appropriate blood tests are carried out, blood pressure readings are up to date, and flagging up concerns regarding the patients that they see. They have provided all the physical health checks for patients on the severe mental health register, and next year we will be extending the service to patients with learning difficulties.

Professional development and career planning from different perspectives

Employer's perspective

There are various ways in which staff may wish to move forward, and good employers can help to introduce career diversity and satisfaction even if staff remain within one practice. The importance of individual performance should be reviewed in order to maximise motivation and achieve optimal results. Employers could use the force-field technique to take an overview of their system and processes for career development for the staff whom they employ. Investing in development opportunities for a good HCA or GPN will bring untold benefits to the practice through new knowledge and skills as well as loyalty and commitment from individuals.

Strategic perspective

There has been a lack of career structure within nursing in general practice, but this is now changing. As HCAs establish a role in general practice, the value of skill mix in practices is becoming apparent. The concept of the Knowledge and Skills Framework and the Skills Escalator should be applied to nurses working in general practice to enable them to take advantage of educational opportunities after identifying specific goals within their annual appraisals. Many nurses in general practice may lack career guidance from within an individual practice. The PCT could provide this together with professional leadership.

Patient's perspective

Nurses working in general practice can move from one role to another more senior role as their careers progress. It is therefore important that patients should consider giving constructive feedback to help career progression for these nurses. Patients will increasingly encounter HCAs in general practice who will perform a variety of basic tasks.

Educationalist's perspective

A variety of career opportunities exist within general practice for nurses. This provides the opportunity for educationalists to consider whether the current range of courses that they provide is sufficient, or whether teaching to increase the range of skills is needed. Education providers need to recognise that continuing professional development is required at a variety of levels, and that updates on clinically related topics are highly valued. Education that provides assessment of competence may be particularly welcomed.

Summary

- The value of paying attention to the future direction of careers is frequently overlooked, but can bring valuable rewards.
- Professional development should be systematically linked to career objectives in order to facilitate progression.
- Mentorship can be helpful in clarifying objectives and keeping continuing professional development on track.

References

1 Schein E. *Career Anchors: discovering your real values.* Oxford: Pfeiffer; 1996.

2 Chambers R, editor. *Career Planning for Everyone in the NHS. The toolkit.* Oxford: Radcliffe Publishing; 2005.

3 Chambers R, Mohanna K, Wakley G *et al. Demonstrating Your Competence 1: healthcare teaching.* Oxford: Radcliffe Publishing; 2004.

4 Garcarz W. *Career Planning for GP Tutors.* Birmingham: 4 Health Limited; 2004; www.4-health.biz

5 Learndirect. *Discover your Hidden Talents.* Milton Keynes: Open University Press; 2003.

6 Chambers R, Tavabie A, Mohanna K *et al. The Good Appraisal Toolkit for Primary Care.* Oxford: Radcliffe Publishing; 2004.

7 Chambers R, Wakley G, Field S *et al. Appraisal for the Apprehensive.* Oxford: Radcliffe Medical Press; 2003.

8 Chambers R, Mohanna K, Wakley G *et al. Demonstrating your Competence as a Healthcare Teacher.* Oxford: Radcliffe Publishing; 2004.

9 Bayley H, Chambers R, Donovan C. *The Good Mentoring Toolkit for Healthcare.* Oxford: Radcliffe Publishing; 2004.

10 Department of Health. *A Review of Continuing Professional Development in General Practice: a Report by the Chief Medical Officer.* London: Department of Health; 1998.

11 Department of Health. *A First Class Service: quality in the New NHS.* London: Department of Health; 1998.

12 Department of Health. *The NHS Knowledge and Skills Framework.* London: Department of Health; 2004.

13 Department of Health. *Agenda for Change: what will it mean for you?* London: Department of Health; 2004.

14   Nursing and Midwifery Council (NMC). *Code of Professional Conduct.* London: NMC; 2004.

15   Department of Health. *Investing in General Practice: the new General Medical Services contract.* London: Department of Health; 2003.

16   Department of Health. *The NHS Plan: a plan for investment, a plan for reform.* London: Department of Health; 2000.

17   Department of Health. *Practitioners with Special Interests in Primary Care: implementing a scheme for nurses with special interests in primary care.* London: Department of Health; 2003.

18   UNISON Open College. *A Professional Profile for Healthcare and Nursing Assistants.* London: Emap Healthcare Ltd; 2004.

19   National Qualifications Framework; www.qca.org.uk/493.html

20   Skills for Health Career Framework; www.skillsforhealth.org.uk/careersframework

6

Working together: integration of nurses and health care assistants working in general practice with other health care professionals

This chapter looks at the advantages of closer integration between general practice nurses and HCAs and other community health care staff. It highlights how this can be achieved and how it can contribute to the delivery of enhanced services. The advantages of a united nursing approach for the purpose of practice-based commissioning are discussed, and the benefits of sharing nurses' knowledge and skills to improve the standard and effectiveness of patient care are emphasised.

Contents

Introduction

Staff who work in general practice represent just one component of the community health care workforce. Patients may also receive care from other sources across the wider primary care trust (PCT), including district nurses, health visitors, school nurses, community matrons, community psychiatric nurses, clinical nurse specialists; allied health professionals and health care assistants, as well as voluntary agencies.

National guidance from the Department of Health[1] emphasises the importance of community nurses working collaboratively with other health care professionals, and eliminating professional boundaries in order to provide the most effective care.

If nurses in general practice do not actively link with other community nurses, there is a real danger that work within the practice will increase unnecessarily because the skills of others are not being used appropriately. GPs are not NHS employees, but independent contractors to the NHS, and they can be viewed as having their own agenda and targets by community nurses who work for the PCT. However, it is essential for everyone to work together. Anyone who works in or for the NHS knows that there is plenty of work out there for everyone.

It is a question of working together as a team so that everyone – the nurses, the patients and the practice – benefits from the right person providing care at the right time.

The GMS contract[2] places emphasis on improving quality of care for patients with long-term conditions. These patients may be receiving care from the practice, other community nurses, social workers or carers from independent or voluntary organisations. This care needs to be coordinated by the practice so that all health care professionals involved with a patient communicate together and are aware of each other's contribution, rather than working in isolation.

Our Health, Our Care, Our Say[3] promotes better partnership working with all stakeholders, including local authorities, to deliver more effective services.

Working with primary care trusts

Nurses in general practice are often able to implement new ideas more quickly than their community nursing colleagues because they work in much smaller and less unwieldy organisations than the PCT. Yet on the other hand PCT-employed community nurses tend to have better support systems than nurses in general practice, with protection against legislation arising from a plethora of PCT policies and procedures. Working in partnership with other health care professionals and related organisations is vital for practices to achieve effective services for patients, but it is important to recognise that joint working must adhere to PCT policies. For example, if practice nurses and district nurses set up a joint wound management clinic, there may be existing PCT policies on wound care that need to be adhered to. Other branches of community nursing are usually more coordinated than general practice nursing because they have a shared management structure that makes communication among nurses easier, and support is therefore more readily available.

Membership of the Professional Executive Committee

Practice nurses are eligible to become nominated members of the Professional Executive Committee (PEC) for the PCT. A place on this board provides an opportunity to represent other practice nursing views and to feed strategic planning and information back to other nurses in general practice.

> Consider becoming part of the PEC if you want to influence PCT practice and help to inform the PCT about life from the perspective of nurses in general practice.

PEC board members campaign for election and are voted in for a 3-year period. PEC activities are additional to normal clinical work, but practices are obliged to give time off for these activities. Typically this will relate to two or three days per month. Although initially it may seem daunting to take on this type of role, PCTs will provide some training or a development programme to support nurse PEC members, who will then have the satisfaction of knowing that they are helping to influence policy and also making the voice of nurses in general practice heard.

Critical success factors for improving integration

In order for health care professionals in general practice to work more closely together, there are certain key principles which need to be emphasised.

Commitment

It is essential that people are really committed to the idea of working with each other to widen the use of skills in the practice team. It is easy to talk about integration, but without commitment, it is all too easy for individuals to continue working in their own professional groups. Key people who need to be committed to making staff work in a more united way are the GP, the general practice nurse(s), the community nurse manager, and team leaders in the community nursing team. It is worth making an effort to convince these people of the benefits of working more closely together before introducing team meetings or information-sharing sessions.

Flexibility and openness

Being flexible about how a team can work together more effectively is essential. Trying to impose an unpopular model, such as weekly meetings, is unlikely to realise any of the potential benefits of teamworking if some individuals don't agree. Openness is also very important. If people have any reason to feel that motives are being hidden, or that information is only being shared selectively, they will resist attempts at integration. Bear in mind that openness may be uncomfortable. If members of the team have different employers, such as the district nurse being employed by the PCT and the general practice nurse being employed by the practice, they are likely to find that their salary level, terms and conditions, and other important factors may be different. Acknowledging such disparities, and the feelings that they may evoke – whether or not there is anything that can be done about the situation – is part of the openness that a team needs in order to work effectively together.

Proactive information sharing

This means that everyone in the team makes a positive effort to ensure that other team members are aware of and can access key information. For example, simply saying that community nurses can 'use' the practice's patient records is meaningless if they are unable to use the practice computer because they don't have passwords. Having a password is of no help if there are so few terminals that district nurses never have the opportunity to enter or retrieve data. This is where the commitment is demonstrated – it may mean rearranging rooms, changing clinic schedules, sharing computers or creating new workstations in order to convert the rhetoric of shared records into reality. Being proactive about sharing other information may mean:

- agreeing regular practice meetings that fit in with community nurses' schedules
- obtaining extra copies of newsletters or circulars so that every team member can have one

- putting up a shared noticeboard so that fliers for educational events are visible to all
- including all team members on 'all staff' email lists
- giving all team members their own 'pigeonhole' for post.

Investing in relationships

Improving relationships across different disciplines or branches of nursing takes effort, time, energy and persistence, in order to create and maintain the team. The investment required may be financial, although it need not be great. Providing extra copies of papers, tea and coffee for meetings, and a noticeboard is not expensive, but all of these things convey the message that this is one team and its members are valued. Just as important is the investment of time. This may be time for team activities (e.g. meetings, away-days, birthday lunches, Christmas dinner) or – more subtle but just as important – informal time. This is the unplanned time for pausing in the corridor to speak to someone, sitting down for a sandwich as a group rather than staying by desks, or listening to someone who has had a difficult encounter with a patient. All team members, not just a nominal team leader or coordinator, need to invest in the team in these ways.

Mutual understanding and respect

This won't just happen automatically, but should arise out of the above-mentioned four factors. By spending time with other team members, sharing each other's information, meeting regularly and talking openly, people develop a broader perspective, and an understanding of each other's roles, challenges and personalities. Trust within the practice is built on the demonstration of respect between members. Listening carefully, maintaining confidences when asked to do so, responding constructively and providing help, or signposts to help, are key ways to demonstrate respect for others.

Improving integration with other community nurses: health care assistants

As an HCA who works in general practice, you can provide an important link between practice staff and other community nurses.

An example of this is the 'one-stop clinic.'

Within a general practice an integrated team can provide a 'one-stop' service for a child health clinic.

- The HCA measures the weight, height and head circumference of the babies and children attending, and ensures that the recording and recall for developmental checks and immunisations are done.
- The GP performs physical and developmental examinations.
- The health visitor gives advice on nutrition, child care and behaviour management.
- The general practice nurse gives immunisations to children and parents.

You might be asked to set up or clear away clinics for dressings or child-hood immunisations. These clinics may be run by district nurses or health visitors who are based elsewhere and just attend the practice to carry out these specific activities. Having a friendly approach and learning more about what they are doing can help these nurses to feel part of a team, rather than visitors to the practice.

In your role as an HCA, you may be involved in creating health promo-tion displays for the waiting room, and you might want to give health professionals attached to the practice your plan for a different display each month. For example, if you are setting up a display about smoking cessa-tion, the local pharmacist may be keen to advertise the availability of nicotine replacement therapy at the same time. Similarly, the health visitor may want to target smoking cessation advice within her interventions while the display is on at the surgery.

Use Tool 6.1 to identify who has special interests in the topics you are highlighting on the practice noticeboard.

You could then ask them to:

• contribute to the display
• advertise the display to the patients they meet
• give you ideas to develop resources.

Improving integration with other community nurses: general practice nurses

The advantages of working more closely with other nurses are both practi-cal and professional.

Access to resources

From a purely practical perspective, widening the group of nurses who act as part of the practice team brings access to greater resources.

• Community nurses will have access to equipment, training events and information through their employing trust that nurses in general practice may not have.
• Nurses in general practice may often have access to a library, GP and nursing journals and circulars, rooms and equipment that the commu-nity nurses do not have.

Thus by working more closely together, each stands to gain something practical from the other.

Managing patient care

Working together also reduces duplication of effort.

• A district nurse may complete an episode of care for a patient instead of leaving some aspects of it to the practice nurse.

- Combining a clinic with a practice nurse and a health visitor can avoid each of them unwittingly seeing the same parent separately.
- With regard to strategic planning for the practice, carrying out health needs assessment on the patient population, identifying patients for registers of chronic disease or undertaking audits, the information already held by the community nurses can save a practice weeks of work.

Professional benefits

The professional benefits of working closely together are no less compelling.

- Functioning as a team allows all members to make the best use of their professional skills and interests, by providing different viewpoints and knowledge of particular conditions, patient groups or services, instead of having to do a bit of everything.
- Working more closely with other health care professionals also provides a wider network of professional support to all involved. Practice nurses frequently report feeling isolated as a nurse in a practice of doctors, and even in practices that have two or three practice nurses, you may find it difficult to provide objective support for each other. In a wider team, there is more likely to be a colleague with whom you can share ideas or concerns, or simply someone who can act as a signpost to a source of information or evidence.
- A wider team also provides a larger pool of expertise to tap into, making it more likely that someone will have relevant experience to bring to bear.
- Liaising with other community nurses more actively may also draw attention to new training and education opportunities.

Nurses who think of themselves as part of a wider team, rather than being limited to the confines of the practice, will find that they have access to more resources, information and opportunities.

Working as part of a team

Making appropriate use of skills within a team that includes the patient as a member will encourage the development of care pathways that cross professional boundaries and prevent people from becoming isolated. This will undoubtedly lead to improved patient care in a cost-effective manner.

A starting point for developing greater integration is to consider exactly who is involved in the wider practice team, and to gain some knowledge of the varied skills available. The wider team is likely to include allied health professionals, pharmacists, social workers, midwives, district nurses, health visitors, school nurses, community mental health nurses and many others. Tool 6.1 provides a record to show who is in the wider practice team, how to contact them, what days they work, and any particular skills or interests they may have.

Tool 6.1 Recording skills in the wider practice team

Add as many rows as you need to the chart below in order to embrace everyone who has direct patient contact with the practice population. Pass it on to your colleagues to collect all the relevant information and then, once it has been returned to you, circulate the completed document to everyone.

Name:

Designation:
Phone number:
Email address:
Days worked:
Special interests or skills:

For example:

Senior practice nurse
Mon, Thurs, Fri
Management of minor illness, and promoting self-care; family planning; asthma
care

HCA
9–12.30 Mon-Fri
Phlebotomy, new patient checks

It is easy to think of community nurses as working only in traditional roles (e.g. the health visitor who works with parents and young children, the district nurse whose caseload consists of housebound older people), without realising that they have more to offer than these core elements of their job. Many individuals have more than the basic skills required to do their job, and an effective team will harness all of these skills.

Case study

Maria has worked as a practice nurse for five years. She works for a large practice with nine GPs, and there are three other practice nurses (all parttime). The practice is housed in a modern purpose-built health centre, and the wider primary care team consists of district nurses, health visitors, school nurses, midwives and community mental health nurses. These staff are all employed by the PCT, which rents the upstairs half of the building. This makes it easier for everyone to work together and not create boundaries.

Maria has always been a friendly outgoing character and feels that she integrates very well with all the health care professionals attached to the practice. She has worked particularly closely with Heather, the community psychiatric nurse, and together they have established a successful stress management group for patients who present with symptoms of anxiety. However, the future of this group is looking uncertain as Heather is leaving the practice, and her replacement will not be in post for several months.

Maria discusses the situation with the GPs, who agree that running this demanding group on her own is probably not a good idea. Maria therefore writes a short article in the practice newsletter explaining that this group will have to close. She is soon contacted by Angela, a district nurse who has been based at the practice for 10 years. She asks Maria why she didn't ask for her help in running the stress management group. Maria replies that she hadn't really thought that a district nurse would be particularly interested in this aspect of care. Angela then explains that she has had a longstanding interest in this area and has recently completed a degree in psychology with a dissertation on the benefits of group therapy for stress management. Angela has also initiated work in the community for housebound patients with long-term conditions who suffer from stress-related symptoms. Maria is shocked that neither she nor any of the GPs knew about this.

This encounter makes her realise how little she knew about the rest of the team of community nurses and their special interests and expertise. She gladly welcomes Angela's help in running the stress management clinic, and resolves to begin a skills directory in which anyone based at the health centre can enter their areas of special interest or expertise.

Collecting information on each other's roles does not have to be a complex or formal process. It can be as simple as asking everyone to write a list, or having a discussion at a team meeting. However, it is useful to record this for any new members who may join the team. It is worth systematically exploring each person's qualifications and professional and life experience, to see how they could contribute in different ways to the services that are provided. Identification of informal or ad-hoc skills could also be included. The ability to carry out an audit, group facilitation skills, or good knowledge of computer programs may not appear on a person's list of formal qualifications, but may still be extremely useful to the team.

Use Tool 6.2 to record the various skills that exist within the wider practice team.

Tool 6.2 Skills audit matrix

This tool will need to be adapted to meet the needs of your particular team. When completing the matrix, remember the following points.

- It is not a competition.
- Everyone in the team does not need the same skills.
- Some skills are useful to have in several people, while others may need only one person to make them available.

- Skills can be gained through a qualification, experience, or a combination of both.
- The matrix can highlight missing or depleted skills in the team, and can be used to plan best use of the training budget available.
- It is a starting point for discussion, not an end in itself.

Tick if you have this skill (✓)

SKILLS	Name:	Name:	Name:	Name:	Name:	Name:
Clinical skills						
Immunisation – child						
Immunisation – adult						
Minor injuries						
Contraception						
Minor surgery						
Venepuncture						
Wound dressing						
Burns treatments						
Smoking cessation						
Menopause advice						
Travel health advice/immunisations						
Mental health promotion						
Mental health care – adult						
Mental health care – child						
Child development assessment						
Exercise advice						

	Tick if you have this skill (✓)					
	Name:	Name:	Name:	Name:	Name:	Name:
Joint assessment						
Falls assessment						
Continence advice						
Diagnostic tests (e.g. *Helicobacter*)						
Chaperoning						
Infection control						
Diabetic foot checks						
New patient checks						
Spirometry						
ECG recording						
Supporting practice nurse triage						

Add other clinical skills relevant to your team

Professional skills

Practice teaching						
Assessment						
Preceptorship						
Mentorship						
Group facilitation						
Evaluation						
Audit						
Research						

	Tick if you have this skill (✓)					
	Name:	Name:	Name:	Name:	Name:	Name:
Team leadership						
Report writing						
Presentation skills						
Add other professional skills relevant to your team						
Managerial skills						
Budgeting						
Staff appraisal						
Staff development						
Service/change planning						
Project management						
Objective setting						
Interviewing						
Add other managerial skills relevant to your team						
Other skills						
Use of computerised patient records						
Word processing						
Spreadsheets						
Presentation software						
Summarising medical records						
Stock control (e.g. ordering vaccines)						

There is an increasing range of voluntary and independent organisations that can contribute towards the care of patients within the practice. These should also be considered when determining the local resources available for patients. Although it may be unnecessary to record which individuals are involved in care delivery, it would be valuable to create a local directory of organisations, with detailed information about their potential contribution. Having compiled a list of health care professionals within the wider primary care team, this could now be extended to contribute to the formation of a local directory for shared use between health and social care services.

Tool 6.3 will provide valuable information for health and social care professionals and patients.

Tool 6.3 Directory of useful local organisations

Compiling the following document could be an interesting activity for an HCA, a student assigned to the practice or a receptionist who wants to be better informed about the facilities available for patients. In order to ensure that the details remain accurate, the document should be reviewed each year by a nominated individual using the contact details below to confirm that the activities and information are still correct. Remember to comply with the requirements of the Data Protection Act.[4]

Name of organisation:
Name and contact details of local contact:
Facilities available locally:
Comments:

For example:

MIND
Bob Smith.
E-mail: Tel no.:
Support groups held in church hall every Thursday afternoon for carers of patients with severe mental illness.
Well-established friendly group; also organises social activities and informal care sitting.

Principles of teamwork

The NHS Modernisation Agency Improvement Leaders' Guides[5] provide ideas on teamworking and the stages that a team will go through during its development.

Characteristics of a team

Unified teams have certain characteristics.[6]

- Team members need:
  - defined roles
  - shared work objectives
  - opportunities to interact together to achieve them.

- The group forming the team should:
  - have an organisational identity
  - have a defined function
  - be recognised as a team by others
  - affect change through the performance of its team members.
- Team members are interdependent for the provision of effective services.

The national report *The Effectiveness of Healthcare Teams in the National Health Service*[7] showed that teamworking could deliver innovative and effective health care for patients.

Effective health care teams:

- communicate and integrate well
- show clear leadership with effective team processes
- emphasise quality
- have clear objectives
- have high levels of participation
- hold good-quality meetings
- introduce innovations in patient care associated with a diverse range of skilled people working together, especially in primary care.

Tool 6.4 will help to create a clear picture of teamwork within the practice.

Tool 6.4 Improving teamwork

Send a questionnaire to all members of the wider practice team, including for example health visitors and district nurses, asking them to consider what works well within the practice and what might work better. Their responses should be anonymous so that everyone feels comfortable about expressing their views.

Collate all of the responses into a list and then select a topic that could be discussed at the next practice meeting.

If the practice does not hold regular practice meetings or meetings that involve the wider team, this could be a good place to start.

Remember that once you have asked for this feedback and discussed it at a meeting, it is important that an action occurs, in order to demonstrate that the discussions have been taken seriously. The team is then more likely to respond to future requests.

Things that your team does well:
Things that could be improved:
Action points:
Action completed:

For example:

Holds regular team meetings.

Not everyone has the chance to speak during the meetings.
Ask each member if they have anything else to contribute before moving on to the next item.
24 April 2006.

Things that your team does not do as well:
Suggestions as to how this could be improved:
Action points:
Action completed:

For example:

Do all health care professionals or HCAs have access to the same patient notes?
If records are computerised, does the district nurse have access to a computer or a password?
Discuss this with the practice manager and GP partners and any other relevant individuals.
Agree a practice policy.
Advise all members.
29 May 2006.

Defining characteristics of team members

It is interesting to identify how, within a team, each member will adopt a different team role that best suits their individual personality and style.[8] This has been well researched by the psychologist Dr Meredith Belbin,[9] who has studied teams over a number of years. Belbin identified nine different team roles, as shown below.

People-orientated roles	Action-orientated roles	Cerebral (thinking) roles
Coordinator	Shaper	Plant
Teamworker	Implementer	Monitor-evaluator
Resource investigator	Completer finisher	Specialist

It may be useful to complete the Belbin self-perception inventory (which can be found at www.belbin.com/belbin-team-roles.htm), or to consider encouraging the team members to complete the inventory together.

Each team member makes a valuable contribution to the team. Ideally, each team would have at least nine members, each of whom would naturally adopt one of the nine different team roles. However, this is unlikely to happen in real life, and most people are a mixture of some or all of the Belbin types.

Understanding the different characteristics of the team members will help to ensure that the patient receives help from the right person, with the appropriate knowledge and skills, at the right time.

How to be an effective team

With the increasing demands on the services provided by general practice, new opportunities and challenges are emerging for nurses and HCAs to take on new roles and ways of working. Some particularly innovative teams may consider developing roles that go beyond existing boundaries with a very specific set of responsibilities to meet service needs. For this to work, there needs to be support for the team with the right resources to do the job – or ideas and solutions to obtain those resources!

A team is more likely to function well if team members:

- are clear about their roles and responsibilities
- are clear about the tasks and responsibilities of the team and how every team member contributes to them
- have clear goals and objectives that are regularly monitored
- understand how they need to work with other teams to provide the right service to a high standard
- are clear about leadership roles and responsibilities
- take a real and active interest in each other's development
- are recognised as a team by others.

Tool 6.5 provides hints and tips to strengthen teamworking.

Tool 6.5 Strengthening teamworking

Work as a team to discuss each of the following points in order to identify more clearly how your team works together.

- Does each member of the team have an up-to-date job description? *Look at Chapter 2 or the WiPP website (www.wipp.nhs.uk) for information on developing job descriptions.*
- Is there a plan to show how all the different roles link with or complement each other? *If not, could you draw up a chart to show how all the job roles interact? This will help everyone to see how their contribution fits within the wider approach to care.*
- Is there an identified team leader? *If not, consider developing this role. Remember that the leader does not necessarily have to be the GP.*
- Do you have regular meetings? Are these held within work time? *If not, consider ways in which time could be put aside to develop these.*
- Do the members of your team have a clear understanding of each other's role? *Consider shadowing other members to learn more about what they do.*
- Do you provide support and encouragement for other members of the team? *Consider how you disseminate news of success (e.g. if someone has completed a course) or innovation. Draft a monthly newsletter.*
- Is there a 'buddy' or mentorship scheme within the team? *Maintaining a buddying role may help to relieve stress by encouraging people to talk about their experiences.*

- Do the team members encourage each other to learn and share new skills? *Team meetings could include teaching sessions or bringing back learning points gained from attending courses or conferences.*

Integrating a new member into the practice team

The introduction of a new team member can be an exciting, challenging and daunting time for both new and established team members. The team will need to change in some way before the person or the role becomes fully integrated. This process is not always smooth, but incorporating the suggestions in Tool 6.5 may help to manage the situation.

Closer working through care pathways and practice-based commissioning

In recent years there has been an increasing emphasis on 'care pathways' (or 'patient pathways') as the basis for care and service planning. This means thinking about more than just what happens to the patient with a particular condition or symptom while they are in primary care. It requires mapping out what should happen when they are referred on to secondary care, and maybe on again to tertiary (specialist) care – and also when they come home again and receive further care or follow-up in primary care. Logically such planning should bring together representatives of each of these care settings, and from all of the professions that will have a major input into the patient's care along the pathway, to produce the agreed pathway. It provides the opportunity to review traditional practice and ensure that each step on the pathway is evidence based and consistent across the geographical area.

The advantages of this approach are that:

- all patients receive an equitable service, regardless of where they present or who sees them
- service quality is improved
- all relevant professionals, in all areas of care delivery, share a common understanding of the locally agreed pattern of referral and treatment
- discrepancies in treatment based on individual clinician preferences or beliefs are reduced
- evidence-based and good practice is embedded in service specifications
- new and locum staff have clear pathways to follow when dealing with patients.

Producing or improving a care pathway will involve more than the nursing team. GPs, hospital staff, allied health professionals and sometimes social services staff will also need to be involved in the planning of the pathway. The development of patient pathways can greatly enhance teamwork by making best use of each individual's skills, sharing information and records, and working together both operationally and strategically. These are the essential building blocks for the whole multi-disciplinary team in implementing a patient pathway.

Practice-based commissioning and integrated working

Practice-based commissioning has been introduced as a way of allowing practices (or groups of practices) to be in charge of ordering appropriate health services that are ideally tailored to fit the needs of the local population. It provides opportunities to get the most appropriate care for the local community, but this can only be achieved if all health care professionals work more closely together to ensure that patients' needs are fully considered. Health visitors will bring a more global view of community health needs with their public health perspective, and district nurses will have greater insight into the needs of the long-term sick. Within the practice, the use of computerised Read codes to categorise reasons for consultations will provide a coordinated view of patient needs. Sharing this information and discussing patient requirements in a joint forum with all community nurses, GPs, allied health professionals and general practice nurses will result in a well-rounded approach that will help to make practice-based commissioning successful. Listening to the perspectives of others will help to broaden horizons and ensure that nurses are not just viewing health needs from a single viewpoint. This in turn will mean that more appropriate care is available to more people.

Integration from different perspectives

Employer's perspective

The advantages of improved partnership working have been emphasised in key national directives.[3] GPs have much to gain from ensuring that all community nurses and allied health professionals attached to the practice work in a coordinated way, without duplication of effort. If all available skills are pooled together, then care can be delivered in a more efficient and cost-effective manner. GPs can facilitate this sharing of skills by hosting regular meetings for the wider team to identify patient needs. Encouraging the wider community health team to use practice resources – such as the practice library, computers, disease registers and patient records – will help to provide a united team approach. In addition, GPs may wish to make use of PCT resources for community nurses, such as training days and clinical supervision groups that will provide support and development for practice nurses and HCAs within the practice.

PCT strategic perspective

Every specialism in community nursing can benefit from closer working with practice nurses. School nurses have common ground and a shared clientele with regard to children and adolescents in need of health promotion, advice and support. Health visitors and practice nurses work with the same young families and vulnerable adults. Streamlining the services will reduce duplication, thereby releasing time and resources. Specialist nurses can greatly increase their effectiveness and reach by working in tandem with practice nurses, rather than duplicating visits, records and assessments.

Some PCTs have worked actively to encourage training across the different branches of community nursing in order to create nurses who are truly generic in their skills. Many PCT strategic objectives, including those outlined in *Standards for Better Health*,[10] can be more easily achieved through joint working between community nurses and practice nurses. For example, public health work (e.g. health promotion and information campaigns, immunisation programmes, and work to mitigate risk factors such as smoking or obesity) is best tackled by nurses who have regular contact with patients over a long timescale. Community nurses are ideally placed to carry out these programmes, with their continuous contact with a registered population. Their involvement with whole families, as well as with individuals, enhances their influence on lifestyle change.

Practice nurses are also essential to the delivery of care to people with long-term conditions. They review the bulk of patients who have relatively low levels of need, in contrast to district nurses, who provide more intensive support to fewer patients with greater needs. This complementary approach is the most efficient way to meet the growing demands of these groups.[11] PCTs can provide mutual benefits for practices by offering professional support for nurses in general practice. Access to community nurses' meetings, clinical supervision, journal clubs and training opportunities would be a real benefit, particularly to smaller practices.

Patient's perspective

Patients should be aware of the range of different skills available from the wide range of health care professionals in primary care. This will help them to access the most appropriate individual. Patients have the right to expect that their care will be coordinated so that they do not have to repeat details of the same problem to different individuals, and that information will be passed between professionals to create a well-informed picture for all. This is on the understanding that all patient information is shared confidentially. If a practice team works closely together, patients may need to make fewer visits to the practice, or receive fewer visits at home, because one team member is taking on several different aspects of care, rather than many individuals needing to be involved. Patients with complex needs may benefit from having shared patient-held records whereby all health care professionals can access the same information, but the patient also has ownership of this to provide them with a full understanding of their own care.

Educationalist's perspective

Educationalists are in a prime position to facilitate closer working relationships between health care professionals, as they are likely to recruit students from different backgrounds who come together to study.

Instead of delivering separate courses that are attractive to particular branches of nursing, educationalists need to create learning experiences that attract diverse members of the health care team. Having a mix of students will add a richness and breadth of perspective to learning. Inter-professional education can be encouraged by creating problem-based scenarios which are analysed and explored by students from a variety of backgrounds.

The trend is towards providing generic education for commonly needed skills, supplemented by specialist education where condition- or pathway-specific knowledge and skills are necessary. This pattern fits with the move away from functional groups – health visitors or practice nurses – towards a more flexible workforce that can accommodate a wider range of entrants, and that can deploy skilled practitioners in non-traditional ways. Some education commissioners have already ceased to commission traditional community nursing courses in favour of this approach. The more students are encouraged to leave their professional groups and learn together, the more likely it is that they will require generic competencies and use each other more appropriately in practice.

Summary

- Nurses working in general practice represent only one aspect of the community health care workforce. They need to work with other health and social care professionals to provide a more comprehensive service.
- Closer partnership working requires effort, but will reap rewards through greater efficiency and the mutual benefits of shared resources.
- Teamworking maximises the use of everyone's skills and avoids duplication of effort.
- Practice-based commissioning will require a global approach to determine patient needs, and this cannot be provided by any single professional group.
- The use of care pathways can help to improve partnership working.

References

1 Department of Health. *Liberating the Talents: helping primary care trusts and nurses to deliver the NHS Plan.* London: Department of Health; 2002.

2 Department of Health. *Investing in General Practice: the new General Medical Services contract.* London: Department of Health; 2003.

3 Department of Health. *Our Health, Our Care, Our Say: a new direction for community services.* London: Department of Health; 2006.

4 *Data Protection Act 1998.* London: HMSO; 1998.

5 *NHS Modernisation Agency Improvement Leaders' Guides*; www.modern.nhs.uk/ improvementguides

6 Arthur H, Wall D, Halligan A. Team resource management: a programme for troubled teams. *Clin Governance Int J.* 2003; **8**: 86–91; www.cgsupport.nhs.uk/PDFs/articles/Team_Resource_Management.pdf

7   Borrill C, Carletta J, Carter AJ *et al. The Effectiveness of Healthcare Teams in the National Health Service. Final report.* London: Department of Health; 2000.

8   Chambers R, Tavabie A, Mohanna K *et al. The Good Appraisal Toolkit for Primary Care.* Oxford: Radcliffe Publishing; 2004.

9   Belbin RM. *Team Roles at Work.* Oxford: Butterworth Heinemann; 2003.

10 Department of Health. *Standards for Better Health.* London: Department of Health; 2004.

11 Department of Health. *Supporting People with Long-Term Conditions: liberating the talents of nurses who care for people with long-term conditions.* London: Department of Health; 2005.

7

Quality improvement and evaluating practice

This chapter highlights the importance of monitoring and measuring quality within general practice. It provides tools for implementing quality checks within practice, and uses the seven pillars of clinical governance to explore all the relevant areas for attention within general practice care when considering quality improvement. The importance of evaluation in order to determine levels of effectiveness is emphasised.

Introduction

Quality is now at the heart of the NHS agenda, and has received due prominence in the GMS contract.[1] Nurses who work in general practice and strive to deliver and maintain the very highest standards should consider their care within the context of the whole practice team. In order to review practice standards, it is helpful to use the Healthcare Commission's *Standards for Better Health*.[2] These are based on the seven pillars of clinical governance,[3] and include the following areas.

- **Safety** – risk management to understand, monitor and minimise the risks to patients and staff and learn from mistakes.
- **Clinical care and cost-effectiveness** – to ensure that the approaches and treatments used are based on the best available evidence.
- **Governance arrangements** – to ensure that systems and audit are in place to collect and interpret clinical information and monitor the quality of patient care.
- **Patient-focused services** – to enable patients and patient organisations to have a say in their own treatment and in the way that services are provided.
- **Accessible and responsive care** – delivery of care by the right person at the right time.
- **Care environment and amenities** – adequate resources that include the recruitment, management and development of staff. This includes the promotion of good working conditions and effective methods of working.
- **Public health** – emphasis on health care that is linked to population needs in order to benefit whole communities.

Resources for quality improvement

Quality improvement can only be achieved by input from a wide range of sources – including individuals from within the practice, but also extending to a number of NHS and Department of Health organisations. The role of all the following organisations which play a key role in quality improvement should be considered, as these can provide useful resources and ideas. See Fig 7.1

- **The National Patient Safety Agency (NPSA)** (www.npsa.nhs.uk) – explores how to make the NHS safer for patients, and encourages examination of sources of error.
- **National Institute for Health and Clinical Excellence** (www.nice.org.uk) – evaluates treatments and management in order to try to establish the most cost-effective care.
- **Healthcare Commission** (www.healthcarecommission.org.uk) – an independent watchdog that reports to Parliament on the performance of NHS trusts in England and Wales.
- **NHS Institute for Innovation and Improvement** (www.institute.nhs.uk) – has expertise in service transformation, technology and product innovation, leadership development and learning. Many of the learning programmes and outputs from previous organisations such as the Modernisation Agency, the NHSU and the National PCT Development Team (NatPaCT) have been subsumed within this organisation.
- **Clinical Governance Support Team** (www.cgsupport.nhs.uk) – supports clinical governance developments.
- **National Primary Care Development Team** (www.npdt.org) – works nationally and regionally to improve care that includes access and coronary heart disease care.
- **National Audit Office (NAO)** (www.nao.org.uk) – scrutinises public spending on behalf of Parliament. It is currently reviewing the implementation of clinical governance within PCTs.
- **Audit Commission** (www.audit-commission.gov.uk) – an independent public body responsible for ensuring that public money is spent economically, efficiently and effectively in health and other areas. Its mission is to be a driving force in the improvement of public services, promoting good practice and helping to achieve better outcomes.

Figure 7.1 Organisations linked to quality improvement

The seven pillars of clinical governance

1 Risk management

Minimising risks to patients and raising awareness of unsafe practice should be an integral component of good practice. Ways of supporting this include:

- completing a skills-based assessment tool which will ensure that the competences of all HCAs and practice nurses are recorded. This will clarify what everyone in the practice is able to do
- reviewing whether induction programmes for new or locum nursing staff are adequate – do they include everything that is needed?
- setting up a system to ensure that 'near-miss' incidents are reported and acted upon

- setting up sessions with other nurses and HCAs in general practice or for the whole practice team to analyse significant events.

Case study: Identifying 'near-miss' incidents

Sue is an experienced practice nurse, but has recently moved practices. She has been at the new practice for about 6 weeks, and is just getting to know some of the patients. She is almost at the end of running a flu clinic. She has already vaccinated 15 patients (mainly elderly, but with a few younger asthmatic patients in between). She calls through her final patient, Mary Smith. Mary, who is 25 years old, comes in saying 'I'm here for my injection. The receptionist said you'd fit me in at the end of the clinic.' Sue draws up the flu injection and has a quick glance at Mary's notes. She notices that she is on repeat medication for a salbutamol inhaler, so assumes that she is attending for the flu injection because of her vulnerability as an asthmatic. Sue is just about to give the injection when she remembers to check whether Mary is pregnant before proceeding. Mary's answer is 'Well, there'd be something wrong with your injections if I was.' This makes Sue stop in her tracks, and she asks Mary what she means. Mary explains that the injection is supposed to be almost 100% effective in preventing pregnancy. Sue realises with horror that Mary has attended for her regular contraceptive injection (Depo Provera), not the flu injection. The receptionist squeezed her in at the end of the flu clinic because there was a vacant slot and she needed to have the injection today. No harm is done, as Sue has not given the injection and is able to remedy the situation.

There is a lot to learn from this case study in terms of the need for systems and processes to prevent this 'near-miss' occurring again. However, the individuals involved often feel upset or embarrassed by their 'near miss', and therefore don't discuss it widely. Having an anonymised reporting system for 'near misses' will bring these incidents into the open so that changes can be made to prevent future risks. Tool 7.1 suggests a simple way of learning from such incidents.

Tool 7.1 Learning from potentially dangerous situations

- Set up one-hour meetings every six weeks or so for the whole practice team to discuss any 'near-miss' incidents that have occurred. Make sure that all GPs, nurses, HCAs and reception staff are invited, as they will all have something to contribute.
- Send out a circular to all practice staff explaining what you are trying to achieve and how learning from mistakes (or near mistakes) will enhance future patient safety. Explain that the system you are setting up will be anonymised so that no individuals can be identified.
- Draft a form to be sent out electronically to all practice staff. Explain that if it is completed electronically, handwriting won't be identifiable. Use headings such as:
    - What was the situation that worried you or almost resulted in a big mistake?

- What did you do about it (if anything)?
- Is there anything you can think of that could prevent this happening again?

- Set up a 'near-misses' incident box somewhere private (e.g. in the staffroom) for completed forms.
- Collect the forms on the day of the meeting and discuss them with all staff members, using the meeting to analyse what happened in the near-miss incidents and how such situations could be prevented from occurring again.
- At the next meeting, start by checking that things which were agreed at the last meeting have now been put in place.
- Hold these meetings regularly. You may want to complete a form yourself relating to a past incident, at least for the first meeting, to make sure that the process takes off. Once people get used to this idea they will contribute as they see what can be learned, and the culture within the practice will gradually become more open.

2 Clinical effectiveness

The following suggestions will help to improve clinical effectiveness within practice.

- Set up meetings with HCAs, nurses and GPs to look at the practice's clinical guidelines and protocols. Ensure that the latest versions are all gathered together for the meeting. They can then be reviewed and updated in a forum where everyone is able to comment and have their say. All protocols should be linked to national guidelines or based on robust evidence.
- Keep all practice policies together in an accessible folder so that any new or locum staff will have easy access to them.
- Make evidence-based information easily accessible. This could be achieved by starting a small 'library' of journal articles categorised by clinical topics (e.g. a box of articles relating to diabetes, coronary heart disease, etc.), compiling a list of websites that staff have found particularly useful and making laminated copies of the list to be kept beside every PC with Internet access.

Protocols provide a clear logical structure, and therefore increase confidence in clinical management. In order to create the most appropriate protocols and guidelines, the whole team should be engaged in creating a unique practice set that is customised to the needs and skills within the practice. Alternatively, access the following website that has links to other publications and websites containing protocols and guidelines: www.ir2.ox.ac.uk/bandolier/painres/download/whatis/WhatareClinGuide.pdf.

Examples of national guidelines that provide robust evidence for clinical management include:

- NICE; www.nice.org.uk
- Scottish Intercollegiate Guidelines Network (SIGN); www.sign.ac.uk
- www.eguidelines.co.uk
- Centre for Reviews and Dissemination; www.york.ac.uk/inst/crd.

Using protocols

Advantages

- Provides a framework for complex, specialised sequences of activities.
- Provides increased autonomy with a focus to shape future work.
- Ensures consensus within the PC team.
- Provides legal protection.
- Identifies training needs.
- May facilitate change.

Disadvantages

- Stifles individual care management.
- May reduce the need for qualified staff.
- Requires regular review.
- Compliance by staff may be problematic.
- Restricts clinical discretion.

What constitutes a good protocol?

- Clearly documented lines of accountability.
- Specific referral criteria.
- Clarity.
- Brevity.
- Fit with professional guidelines.

The following website provides examples of over 100 protocols for use in general practice: www.equip.ac.uk/practiceManagement/docs/protocols/protocols.htm.

3 Education, training and CPD

Appropriate training is essential for the delivery of good-quality, evidence-based care. Registered nurses have a responsibility[4] to ensure that they remain up to date and well informed about their own area of practice. They are also responsible for demonstrating commitment and support to education and training. This means being involved in the development of junior staff, including HCAs. All nurses within general practice should have their competence assessed in order to obtain an objective measure of what individual nurses can and cannot do. The practice is required to provide opportunities for staff development as part of the GMS contract.[1]

The GMS contract[1] (section 4.20) states that 'all practice-employed nurses should be supported to participate in clinical supervision and appraisal.' Clinical supervision is regarded by nursing professional bodies (the NMC and the RCN) as a supportive way to facilitate learning from experience, and should therefore be viewed as an integral component of clinical governance. Clinical supervision is discussed in Chapter 5.

Annual appraisal should take place as part of continuing professional development because it helps to identify individual strengths and weaknesses. It is also helpful to have additional, less formal reviews on a more frequent basis.

For HCAs, these could be conducted by a practice nurse. For practice nurses, it may be appropriate for the GP to review the delivery of clinical care if there is no senior nurse. Appraisal is discussed in Chapter 5.

Improved integration with the wider primary care team can aid education, and may disclose new opportunities for training (*see* Chapter 6). Sharing experiences and skills through networking or local forums can be educational, and using peer review could help to support self-assessment. Tool 3.2 (*see* Chapter 3) provides an example of how this could be successfully implemented.

4 Use of information

The information highway means that it is easier to keep up to date. There are no excuses for ignorance! Connecting for Health[5] promises some real opportunities for the future with the advent of electronic patient records. Over the next 10 years the national programme for IT in the NHS plans to connect more than 30,000 GPs in England to almost 300 hospitals. General practices have introduced computerisation at a varied pace, but it is now viewed as an essential tool for improving efficiency of care.

Within the practice, information about patients is generally entered using Read codes. This makes audit and categorisation of information much easier. Decision-making support software such as PRODIGY[6] can provide evidence-based guidance and information for patient management.

When using electronic patient records, it is essential to ensure that all care plans can be individualised and that alert systems are put in place to identify particular areas or needs.

5 Staffing and staff management

General practice partnerships are often fairly small, but it is still important to have clearly identifiable lines of managerial responsibility. Practice nurses may be asked to act as line managers for junior staff or HCAs. If so, they should be adequately prepared for the role of monitoring staff performance and undertaking appraisals. The GMS contract[1] refers to improved HR services for staff, including entitlement to all NHS conditions and initiatives to 'Improve Working Lives.' Any requests for flexible working should therefore be met with a favourable response so long as the requests are reasonable. Achieving quality care within general practice is all about teamwork, and it pays to value all members of the team. Tool 7.2 provides a way of assessing how well the team members are working together.

Tool 7.2 How well is your team functioning?[7]

Complete the following checklist of how your practice team functions from your perspective as a member of the team.

This is a self-assessment and your perspective might be biased, or you might not know what standards to expect. So it will be best if you compare your answers to

*the questions below with the responses to the same checklist completed by others in
your team, such as your practice manager or the other practice nurses, HCAs or
GPs.*

Please circle your response to each statement:

Usually
Seldom
Not at all
Score:

There is good communication between colleagues at work.

There is good communication between the practice manager and staff.

Team members' functions are clear.

General practice nurses and HCAs are proud to be working in this practice.

Doctors and/or the practice manager generally resolve staff problems.

General practice nurses and HCAs are treated with respect by the GPs,
receptionists and practice manager.

There is a person-friendly culture at work.

There are opportunities for self-improvement.

Positive feedback about performance is the norm at work.

Nurses are well trained for the tasks that they are asked to do.

Team members' responsibilities are clear.

There is good leadership in the practice team.

Score as follows: *Usually = 3, Seldom = 1, Not at all = 0.*

Total:

Conclusion

Scores between 27 and 36: Congratulations, you belong to a well-function-
ing team.

Scores between 26 and 15: You may like to discuss your findings with the
practice manager to see whether any changes can be made to strengthen
teamworking.

Scores of 15 or lower: *This suggests that the team needs to do some develop-ment work so that the team members can function together more effectively. Talk to your line manager about how you could help to move this forward. It may be appro-priate to consider using an external consultant or someone from the PCT to help to facilitate practice team development.*

You cannot do much as one individual to change the culture and quality of the teamworking in your practice. You need to persuade the rest of the team to tackle any problems under the leadership of the practice manager and/or GPs.

Good communication between staff assists in the management of change. Regular meetings with the practice team to discuss clinical issues can be invalu-able in maintaining the highest standards of care. Consider incorporating the following topics within practice meetings:

- interesting clinical cases
- significant events
- in-house training
- changes to the practice formulary
- practice policies.

Attendance at clinical meetings could be improved if the practice creates protected non-appointment time and is prepared to pay overtime to those who come in specially to attend.

6 Clinical audit

Audit is the method used 'to assess, evaluate and improve the care of patients in a systematic way, to enhance their health and quality of life.'[8] It is a reliable way of determining whether the services that are being delivered are effective. Audit can be surprisingly simple to undertake, and should be considered an essential element of health care practice. Audit measures performance against a defined standard to find out whether a service is as good as it should be. All nurses working in general practice should be involved in the audit process to some extent. The level of involvement may vary from designing and conduct-ing the audit to contributing to data collection or commenting on the standard that is set as best practice.

Clinical audit should also include all the non-clinical components of service provision. The standards of clinical care in general practice cannot be measured without looking at access to and availability of care, and the effectiveness of systems. Everyone in the practice team contributes to this. Staff in general practice can only operate effectively if they work in a well-connected way with the wider community health care team and local hospitals.

The main steps of the audit cycle are as follows.

- Prioritise and select the topic of your audit, working with others in your team or practice.
- Set objectives relating to the reason(s) why the audit is being carried out.

- Review the literature for that topic and agree the criteria and standards that you think are reasonable.
- Design the way in which you will conduct the audit.
- Collect the data and analyse them.
- Feed back the findings. Meet with colleagues or your team to discuss the findings and determine the reasons for the satisfactory or disappointing results.
- Make a timetabled action plan to implement any changes that are needed.
- Review your standards. You might keep the standards you previously set, or drop the standards if the initial thinking was unrealistic, or raise them if the previous standards were not challenging enough.
- Re-audit, creating improvements and then successive audit cycles.

Questionnaires are frequently used within an audit to gauge the opinion of patients or health care professionals. The wording of the questions is all-important,[10] so note the following key points.

- Use simple language.
- Be consistent.
- Do not assume common knowledge.

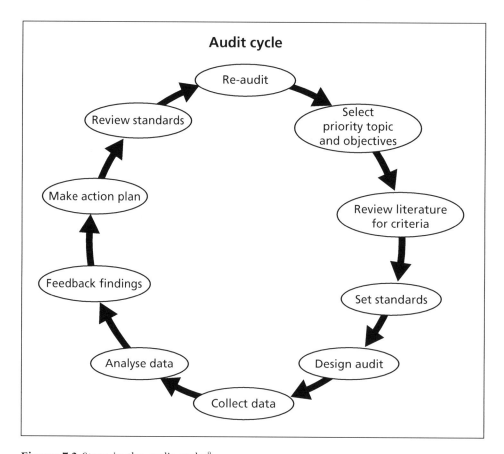

Figure 7.2 Steps in the audit cycle.[9]

- Avoid using leading questions.
- Avoid using questions that have two parts.
- Be aware of the social desirability effect, whereby answers can be given to try to please whoever has set the questionnaire.
- Take care when using questions referring to time.
- Collect only essential data.
- Think carefully about the type of questions to use.
- Collect data only on subjects that you can do something about.

Another way of ensuring that best practice is measured is to use the benchmarking process outlined in *Essence of Care*[11] (www.dh.gov.uk/assetRoot/04/12/79/15/04127915.pdf).

7 Patient/service user and public involvement

The increasing emphasis on patient and public involvement in the delivery and planning of services is clearly indicated within *The NHS Plan*.[12] The intention is to involve and consult patients and the general public about key issues within the NHS, such as identifying local needs and priorities and evaluating the quality of services from a patient satisfaction perspective. The opinions of patients within a practice should be sought prior to implementation of change (e.g. via the Patient Advice and Liaison Service [PALS] or the practice patients' committee).

Tool 7.3 provides some ideas on how to gain insight into the patient perspective.

Tool 7.3 Identifying what patients think about the practice

As a practice nurse or HCA you may feel that you know whether patients get on well with you or not, but this is a subjective matter and may be linked to your personality rather than to the service you deliver. If you undertake regular patient satisfaction surveys you will have a more robust method of determining patients' views.

- Ask patients about the service you provide, but be careful not to use questions that are based on your values and assumptions as a health care professional. Simply providing blank forms or asking open-ended questions is likely to provide a more accurate reflection of what the service is really like for patients.
- If you want to conduct a patient satisfaction survey, consider using a validated tool that has been demonstrated to yield meaningful results. An example of this is the General Practice Assessment Survey[13] (www.gpaq.info). Some validated tools may incur costs, but consider whether the benefits to the practice (and not having to spend time and effort drafting your own survey) are worthwhile.
- If you want to know more about what matters to patients in general practice, read the Department of Health's *National Survey of NHS patients: General Practice*[14] or articles based on this.[15] They cover a wide range of issues, including access, waiting times, views of GPs and practice staff, and the quality and range of services in general practice.

Evaluating practice

If evaluation is not undertaken, it will be impossible to determine whether efforts have been worthwhile, or if care needs to be delivered in different ways. Incorporating evaluation into every aspect of work in general practice will help to ensure high-quality standards and demonstrate a desire to seek continual improvement. Evaluation should be considered from a variety of perspectives in order to make it meaningful, and is a vital component of quality assurance. However, it should be kept as simple as possible in order to avoid wasting resources on unnecessary bureaucracy.[16]

If evaluation is to be effective, it should be:

- efficient, effective and economical – taking into account the costs and effectiveness of what is being evaluated, as well as the evaluation process itself
- valid – measuring what it is intended to measure
- reliable – producing accurate findings
- flexible and practical – not burdensome
- fair – not favouring any particular person or group, either directly or indirectly, and including all elements of care
- in proportion – to the specific issues or elements of care
- accountable – linked into any internal or external reports that are part of the accountability structure for individuals, in the practice or in the PCT
- coordinated – with the practice or PCT development or review processes.[2]

Stages of evaluation

There are two phases to evaluation – *formative* and *summative*.

- A formative evaluation involves collecting data during a development and using it to shape what happens according to what problems arise and what seems to be working well.
- A summative evaluation occurs after the activity has ended, and is used to make judgements about the success or otherwise of the development or service that is being evaluated.

One way of approaching evaluation is to set targets and timescales that are realistic for the particular context and issues that are being evaluated.

Tool 7.4 provides some hints and tips for good practice.

Tool 7.4 Achieving meaningful evaluation

- Specify exactly what you want to evaluate and what you hope to achieve (e.g. to evaluate the effectiveness of the HCA role).
- Break down the overall objective into measurable components (e.g. the HCA role in effective delivery, efficiency and patient care experience related to coronary heart disease).
- Set priorities against what you need to achieve – for example:

- to ensure that all patients are being recalled at appropriate times by the HCA
- to ensure that patient screening is recorded appropriately
- to ensure that patients are satisfied with the service.

- List the time and resources involved (e.g. is a computerised system in place to identify recall or will a manual search be required?).
- Obtain agreement from the practice team as to how the evaluation will be carried out (e.g. will manual or computerised searching of records be utilised? Will patient questionnaires be used?).
- Describe the expected impact of the activity and who will be affected (e.g. the efficiency of the HCA role in recall of patients can be measured).
- Determine how long the evaluation will take overall, and how the results will be recorded and disseminated (e.g. will the results be discussed at a practice meeting?).
- Review and refine the objectives of the evaluation and check that the evaluation has achieved those objectives.

Evaluating the aspects of care that are most highly valued by patients ensures that the practice is always patient focused. Issues that are important to patients may include:

- availability and accessibility – including appointments, waiting times, physical access and telephone access
- technical competence – including the knowledge and skills of HCAs, and the effectiveness of the treatments that they provide
- communication skills – including providing time, exploring patients' needs, listening, explaining and giving information.
- interpersonal attributes – including humane, caring attitude, supportiveness and trust.
- organisation of care – including continuity of care, coordination of care and availability of on-site services.

The whole practice team needs to be involved in evaluating the work that is undertaken within the practice. Evaluation should look at the structure, process and outcome of work. This can also be interpreted as the 'What', 'How' and 'Outcome' relating to services delivered. Evaluation should become a routine part of work, and may be made easier by using the same headings for all services, as this will aid comparison. Consider the following way of structuring evaluation.

- Record what actually happened – such as the content of an induction, or the setting up of a diabetic clinic.
- Comment on how it worked out – how well the induction ran, how smoothly the diabetic clinic ran, how many patients were seen, and their comments.
- Discuss the outcome – what was achieved as a result of the induction, any medication changes that were initiated as a result of patients attending the clinic, the consequent improvement in long-term control of individuals' diabetes, the extra attention and education received by patients.

Quality improvement and evaluating practice from different perspectives

Employer's perspective

General practices have achieved high clinical quality scores since the Quality and Outcomes Framework (QOF) and the GMS contract were introduced, which provided financial incentives for high-quality care.

Many of the improvements achieved by meeting the QOF targets have come from structured care provided by nurses in chronic disease management. It is therefore important to consider how quality of care that is delegated to nurses and others within the practice team can be assured within the practice. Success within general practice is largely dependent on teamwork, and paying attention to the nature of the teamwork will reap rewards.

PCT's strategic perspective

PCTs have a responsibility to ensure that GP practices, acting as independent contractors, provide high-quality care. Clinical governance can be used by the PCT to monitor quality and also to identify the priority areas that need development. The Quality Outcomes Framework has introduced a new measure of quality for general practice, with systematic examination of general practice services and standards of care. There are many ways in which PCTs can seek assurance of quality standards within general practice settings, and this needs to be approached in a non-threatening and facilitative manner, with the aim of improved patient care firmly in mind.

Since the introduction of the new GMS contract, GPs have been sharing data about their clinical activities more widely both with each other and with local NHS managers. Nurses in general practice have often had a key role in enabling this to happen. As practice nurses take their professional leadership from within the PCT (which is responsible for clinical governance), even though they may be employed by the practice, they have engaged more readily with the PCT and not perpetuated the 'us and them' culture. Sharing evaluations of practice between general practice and wider community services will help to create the type of seamless care that is required for quality improvements to be consistent and meaningful.

The patient's perspective

Patient opinions are increasingly recognised as being important[15] in helping to raise standards of health care. Patients are likely to find that general practice nurses and HCAs play an increasingly important part in the delivery of their care within general practices. More general practice nurses are taking on advanced roles by running nurse-led clinics where nurses take responsibility for care. Patients may therefore wish to get involved with rating how well the nurses in a practice are providing care. Patients should be encouraged to consider the extent to which nurses:

- give good advice about health consistent with that provided by the doctors and other nurses in the practice team
- are generally helpful and good at listening to problems
- have a respectful, kindly, informative manner
- provide a choice with regard to treatment.

Patients may be reassured to see that their practice surgery has achieved recognised quality standards demonstrated by awards such as Investors in People or a Quality Practice Award. Similarly, patients will appreciate their opinions being sought within patient satisfaction surveys,[14,15] and these can be initiated locally or nationally. Membership of a Patient and Public Involvement (PPI) forum provides patients with the opportunity to comment on all aspects of their care. PPI forums exist within every NHS trust and PCT in England, and consist of local people who have an interest in health services within their local community. They help to raise awareness of the needs and views of patients and the public and the services available to them. Further information can be obtained by visiting www.cppih.org.

The educationalist's perspective

Higher education institutions (HEIs) are familiar with the need to demonstrate quality within their service provision through the HEI Quality Assurance Assessment process. Assisting general practice nurses in demonstrating the quality of their care should be an integral part of any course for GPNs. Education programmes should embed a culture of quality within practice, including the need for evaluation of care in order to ensure that standards are being met. Part of the role of education is to advise on how this process can be introduced in a simple yet effective format.

Although the concept of clinical governance is now mainstream within larger health care organisations, it is sometimes less familiar within small general practices. There is still a need for education and training in the aspects of clinical governance and how the information can be used to improve quality. A selection of courses on clinical governance can be found at www.wisdomnet.co.uk/default.asp, and other advice on a possible curriculum can be found on Royal College of General Practitioners' website (www.rcgp.org.uk/corporate/responses/curriculum/pdfs/Clinical Governance.pdf).

Summary

- Quality is at the heart of the NHS agenda, and has received due attention within the GMS contract and the Quality Outcomes Framework.
- Quality care can only be achieved through a team approach involving both local and national resources.
- Quality improvement can be effectively considered under the seven pillars of clinical governance, namely:
  - risk management

- clinical effectiveness
- education, training and CPD
- use of information
- staffing and staff management
- clinical audit
- patient/service user and public involvement.
• Evaluation is fundamental to quality, and should be an integral part of nursing in general practice.

References

1   Department of Health. *Investing in General Practice: the new General Medical Services contract.* London: Department of Health; 2003; www.doh.gov.uk/gmscontract/thecontract.htm.

2   Healthcare Commission. *Standards for Better Health.* London: Department of Health; 2004.

3   Chambers R, Wakley G. *Making Clinical Governance Work for You.* Oxford: Radcliffe Medical Press; 2000.

4   Nursing and Midwifery Council. *Code of Professional Conduct.* London: Nursing and Midwifery Council; 2002.

5   Connecting for Health. *National Programme for IT in the NHS;* www.connecting forhealth.nhs.uk.

6   PRODIGY. *PRODIGY Knowledge website;* www.prodigy.nhs.uk.

7   Chambers R, Davies M. *What Stress in Primary Care!* London: Royal College of General Practitioners; 1999.

8   Irvine D, Irvine S, editors. *Making Sense of Audit.* Oxford: Radcliffe Medical Press; 1991.

9   Wakley G, Chambers R. *Clinical Audit in Primary Care: demonstrating quality and outcomes.* Oxford: Radcliffe Publishing; 2005.

10 Parsley K, Corrigan P. *Quality Improvement in Healthcare: putting evidence into practice.* 2nd ed. Cheltenham: Stanley Thornes; 1999.

11 NHS Modernisation Agency. *Essence of Care: patient-focused benchmarks for clinical governance.* London: Department of Health. 2003.

12 Department of Health. *The NHS Plan.* London: Department of Health; 2000.

13 Ramsay J, Campbell J, Schoter S *et al.* The General Practice Assessment Survey (GPAS): tests of data quality and measurement properties. *Fam Pract.* 2000; **17:** 372–9.

14 Department of Health. *National Survey of NHS Patients: general practice.* London: Department of Health; 1999; www.dh.gov.uk/assetRoot/04/02/36/11/04023611.pdf.

15 Bower P, Roland M, Campbell J *et al.* Setting standards based on patients' views on access and continuity: secondary analysis of data from the General Practice Assessment Survey. *BMJ.* 2003; **326:** 528–534.

16 Wood L. *Review, Agree, Implement, Demonstrate.* Leicester: National Clinical Governance Support Team; 2001.

Index